OXFORD MEDICAL PUBLICATIONS

ORAL AND DENTAL TRAUMA
IN CHILDREN AND ADOLESCENTS

Oral and Dental Trauma in Children and Adolescents

GRAHAM ROBERTS
Professor of Children's Dentistry,
The Eastman Dental Institute and
The Institute of Child Health,
University of London

AND

PETER LONGHURST
Senior Lecturer/Honorary Consultant,
Department of Orthodontics and Paediatric Dentistry,
Guy's and St Thomas's Medical and Dental School,
University of London

Oxford   New York   Tokyo
OXFORD UNIVERSITY PRESS
1996

Oxford University Press, Walton Street, Oxford OX2 6DP

Oxford   New York
Athens   Auckland   Bangkok   Bombay
Calcutta   Cape Town   Dar es Salaam   Delhi
Florence   Hong Kong   Istanbul   Karachi
Kuala Lumpur   Madras   Madrid   Melbourne
Mexico City   Nairobi   Paris   Singapore
Taipei   Tokyo   Toronto
and associated companies in
Berlin   Ibadan

Oxford is a trade mark of Oxford University Press

Published in the United States
by Oxford University Press Inc., New York

A catalogue record for this book is available from the British Library

Library of Congress Cataloging in Publication Data
ISBN 0 19 262055 X h/b
0 19 262049 5 p/b
Typeset by EXPO Holdings, Malaysia
Printed and bound in Hong Kong

PREFACE

Our involvement in the teaching of the management of oro-dental trauma to undergraduates and general dental practitioners over many years has persuaded us of the need for a concise textbook on this subject. The principal aim of this book, therefore, is to meet this need.

Most children and adolescents who suffer oro-dental injury will be taken, in the first instance, to a general dental practitioner or will be referred there after initial assessment and treatment at a local hospital casualty department. We believe that the majority of these patients can be cared for by the dental practitioner provided that he or she has a sound understanding of the biological basis of the various treatment options. On occasion, the extent and severity of the injuries sustained will necessitate the patient being referred for specialist care. We hope that this text will provide the undergraduate and practitioner alike, with the understanding and confidence to care for these young patients.

No clinician working today in the field of dental traumatology can fail to acknowledge the remarkable contribution made by Professor Jens Andreasen and Dr Frances Andreasen of The Royal Dental College, Copenhagen, Denmark, and their many colleagues and co-workers. Their wealth of experience, backed by careful clinical and laboratory research, has guided their teaching and is a constant inspiration to us all. Our debt to them will be apparent throughout this book and we formally record our thanks.

London   G. J. R.
December 1995   P. L.

ACKNOWLEDGEMENTS

It is a great pleasure to be able to acknowledge the constant stimulus provided by generations of undergraduates, postgraduates, and dental practitioners who have had to endure our teaching of this important topic. Also to acknowledge the encouragement of our colleagues. We thank Dr C. J. Hobbs, Consultant Paediatrician at St James' Infirmary, Leeds, for Fig. 3.1. We are particularly grateful to Miss Sian Roberts for her skilful execution of the line drawings. Finally, we offer our sincere thanks to our families for their forbearance in the production of this book.

CONTENTS

1 The problem, classification, epidemiology, and aetiology

1 The problem, classification, epidemiology, and aetiology

THE PROBLEM

ORO-DENTAL injury in children is a cause of much pain and distress. For the parents of a child damaged in this way the immediate concern is that of obtaining first-class emergency care. Once the acute problems have been successfully dealt with there remains the intermediate and long-term management.

One in ten children suffer injury resulting in significant damage to the oro-dental structures. Incipient malocclusion may be worsened as a result of the trauma and need specialist attention when planning treatment.

The treatment needs resulting from oro-dental injuries are significant. In one group of about 2500 patients with trauma resulting from sports injuries, 52% required conservative restorative treatment, 37% required endodontic treatment, and 41% required crowns or bridges. Only 17% did not require active treatment.

General and specialist dental practitioners caring for the young are, therefore, likely to be faced with many problems associated with oro-dental injury, which can present in infants, children, and adolescents. Trauma may affect the dento-alveolar structures in such a way that treatment will continue at least until the patient has reached maturity and even then the consequences may have a lifelong effect.

The General Dental Practitioner (GDP) needs to be in a position to provide such treatment for the majority of these patients, although some will need the additional care of specialist practitioners. A further small group will need combined orthodontic and paediatric dental care. Notwithstanding specialist treatment, the focal point for the individual patient is the long-term care provided by the GDP.

CLASSIFICATION OF ORO-DENTAL INJURIES

Oro-dental injuries have been classified according to aetiology, pathology, or treatment. The main purpose of such classifications has been to provide clinicians with a straightforward way to identify the damage caused by a traumatic episode and enable the most effective immediate and long-term treatment to be carried out. The following example (after Ellis 1960), has been used for a number of years:

Class I   Fracture of enamel
Class II   Fracture of enamel and dentine
Class III   Fracture of enamel, dentine, and pulp
Class IV   Fracture of the root
Class V   Avulsion

A major limitation of such a classification is that it concentrates mainly on the visible tooth injuries and takes no account of the effect on the pulp or the supporting structures. The authors believe that a descriptive categorization of damage, based on the anatomical distribution of the injuries and their effect on the dento-alveolar tissues, provides a sound biological basis for treatment. The categories of injury draw, inevitably, on the work of many authors but particularly that of Andreasen (1981) and Andreasen and Andreasen (1994). For the sake of clarity, the categories are listed and discussed separately. Nevertheless, many patients present with a combination of injuries, so treatment needs to be planned accordingly.

Crown fracture

1. Fracture involving enamel.
2. Fracture involving enamel and dentine.
3. Simple crown–root fracture involving enamel, dentine, and cementum.
4. Fracture involving enamel, dentine, and pulp.
5. Complicated crown–root fracture involving enamel, dentine, pulp. and cementum.

Root fracture

1. Fracture involving cementum, dentine, and pulp.

Periodontal tissue injury (luxation injury)

1. Concussion.
2. Subluxation (loosening).
3. Lateral luxation.
4. Intrusive luxation (intrusion).
5. Extrusive luxation (extrusion).
6. Avulsion (total luxation).

Pulp and periapical tissue injury

1. Late presentation: non-vital immature tooth with, or without, apical bone loss.

Injury to deciduous dentition and developing permanent teeth

Injury to soft tissues or gingivae

1. Contusion of soft tissues or gingivae.
2. Abrasion of soft tissues or gingivae.
3. Laceration of soft tissues or gingivae.

Injury to the supporting bone

1. Comminution of alveolar socket.
2. Fracture of alveolar wall.
3. Fracture of alveolar process.
4. Fracture of mandible or maxilla.

EPIDEMIOLOGY

A reliable assessment of the distribution of oro-dental injury in the population is extremely difficult. There are two main reasons for this. First, data derived from treatment centres records only those patients who perceive a need for treatment and attend the centre. Many apparently minor injuries will, therefore, go unrecorded. A few of these will develop complications and present late. Secondly, any epidemiological study only records injury which has a visible effect on the teeth. Consequently, many injured teeth (e.g. those with concussion or sub-luxation) will be overlooked. In addition, injuries to the soft tissues and alveolar bone will heal, become invisible and again not be recorded. Data on injuries in child populations must be considered in the light of these difficulties.

PREVALENCE

Prevalence is the number of cases present in a given population at any one time. The larger the number in the sample, the more reliable is the estimate.

While there are many studies on the prevalence of injury to the permanent dentition, there have been few studies of the deciduous dentition. The most representative of these showed that by 7 years of age approximately 30% of children exhibited evidence of trauma to the deciduous dentition (Fig. 1.1). The permanent dentition revealed signs of trauma in over 20% of children in one Scandinavian study (Fig. 1.2). The most comprehensive study on a nation-wide basis is the United Kingdom Children's Dental Health Survey of 1993 in which over 19 000 children were examined; by 15 years of age 26% of children showed signs of trauma to the teeth. When it is remembered that soft tissue and bony damage are unlikely to have been recorded, it is apparent that more than 30% of children will have experienced some oro-dental trauma by the age of 15 (Fig. 1.2).

INCIDENCE

Incidence is the increase in the number of cases over a given period of time. In the deciduous dentition there are approximately 5% of new cases per year. These are not evenly distributed. There is an increase from 1 year of age with a peak of just under 10% by 3 years of age. Most children start to walk at about 1 year of age; by 2 years of age children can run and by 3 years of age, ride a tricycle.

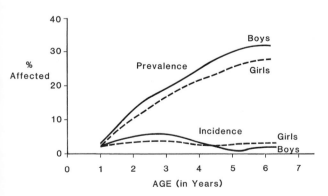

Fig. 1.1 Prevalence and incidence of oro-dental injury in the deciduous dentition. (Redrawn after J. O. Andreasen 1981.)

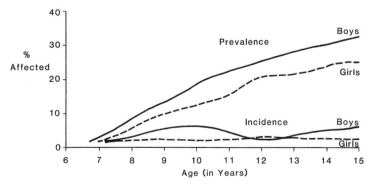

Fig. 1.2 Prevalence and incidence of oro-dental injury in the permanent dentition. (Redrawn after J. O. Andreasen 1981.)

This rapid increase in physical activity, and increasing adventurousness, is associated with an increase in trauma in general and that involving the oro-dental structures in particular.

A similar incidence pattern is seen when the permanent teeth are considered. There is an average incidence of approximately 4% per annum with a peak at 10 years of age (Fig. 1.2). The increased incidence between 8 and 10 years of age is thought to be associated with the more boisterous recreational activities in this age group, coupled with less cautious behaviour.

An important factor in the injuries affecting the permanent dentition is that the peak incidence of injury between the ages of 8 and 11 years means that these injuries affect immature teeth. A common assumption is that by 10–11 years of age, upper permanent incisors have a mature root with a constricted apical foramen. This is rarely true (Friend 1967). Confusion can be caused by the fact that on intra-oral radiographs, which show only the mesio-distal dimension, the root frequently appears mature with a narrow canal and apical constriction. However, at this age the root canal is oval, with an incomplete apical foramen, but as the 'ovality' is bucco-palatal it cannot be seen on the usual intra-oral radiograph. The significance is that such teeth cannot be treated in the same way as mature teeth in older patients, particularly where endodontic therapy is contemplated.

Gender distribution

General studies of oro-dental injury have shown a consistent difference between the sexes, boys being more likely to suffer trauma than girls, in both the deciduous and permanent dentitions (Figs 1.1, 1.2). In some studies, up to twice as many boys as girls suffer trauma to their permanent teeth, although this is not so marked in the deciduous dentition. In the United Kingdom, the Children's Dental Health Survey (1993) showed a male to female ratio of approximately 3:2.

Distribution of injuries

The teeth most commonly damaged are the upper central incisors. The differential susceptibility of individual incisor teeth is 73% for upper centrals, 18% for lower centrals, 6% for lower laterals, and 3% for upper laterals (Fig. 1.3). Other

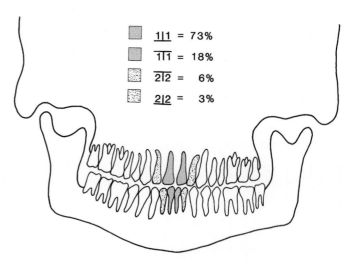

Fig. 1.3 Schematic representation of the relative frequency of injury to different teeth in the permanent dentition. (From Ellis 1960.)

teeth, such as upper and lower canines, represent only a very small proportion of damaged teeth. Upper central incisors are most commonly affected because they are, in general, the most prominent teeth.

Relationship to overjet

The degree of prominence of teeth is an important predisposing factor to oro-dental injury. Children with an overjet of 5 mm or more are 1.5 times more likely to suffer trauma than those with an overjet of less than 5 mm. This difference rises twofold where the overjet is greater than 9 mm.

TYPE OF INJURY

Few investigators have addressed this aspect, but approximate figures may be obtained by combining data from several sources (see Table 1.1). Although the most common injury is probably concussion, it is unlikely to be recorded in many instances as the symptoms may not be severe enough for the patient to seek treatment and signs of the injury do not persist. The most commonly reported injuries are fracture of enamel, fracture of enamel and dentine, and subluxation which, together, constitute over 70% of all recorded oro-dental injuries. The less common injuries—avulsion, root fracture, intrusive and extrusive luxation—are encountered so infrequently that it is difficult for the individual practitioner to become sufficiently adept at confidently managing such problems on the basis of clinical experience alone.

SOCIAL FACTORS

Other, often socially related, factors contribute to oro-dental injury. Most children and young people suffer such injury while running about, playing, participating in organized sport, fighting, and travelling. The majority of injuries affect only a single tooth, but bicycle, and particularly motorcycle and automobile accidents, can cause multiple injuries. Oro-dental injury associated with contact sport is well recognized and can be reduced by the use of mouthguards but, in fact,

Table 1.1 Type of dental injury, by number and percentage, in children 7–16 years of age

Type of injury	No. of teeth	%
Fracture of enamel	1008	54.9
Fracture of enamel and dentine	305	16.6
Fracture of enamel, dentine, and pulp	89	4.8
Fracture of root	16	1.0
Concussion	134	7.3
Subluxation	190	10.4
Luxation	36	1.9
Avulsion	29	1.6
Other injuries	27	1.5
Total	1834	100

Based on data from several sources.

accounts for only a small percentage of these injuries. The incidence of injury increases during the winter months when people are more likely to lose their footing in the ice and snow. It is also recognized that some children appear to be accident-prone, suffering several bouts of trauma to the same tooth/teeth.

Patients with disability

Children with learning difficulty or physical disability have an increased incidence of oro-dental injury, the number of traumatic episodes being related to the type and severity of the condition. The diagnosis and care of injuries may be made more difficult by the special behaviour–management problems some of these children present, compounded by the fact that repeated injury is common in some conditions (e.g. epilepsy and some forms of cerebral palsy).

AETIOLOGY

Oro-dental injury results from a blow to the soft tissues and/or teeth. The blow is often severe, although even apparently trivial blows can have untoward effects. A detailed review of the case histories of a large number of patients reveals a similarly large number of ways in which damage to the face and teeth can be caused. When the aetiology of the injuries is considered, surprisingly few would have been amenable to preventive measures. Nevertheless, the provision of mouth protectors for participants in contact sports is a worthwhile measure.

A convenient way to consider aetiological factors is to relate them to chronological or developmental age.

Preschool years (0–4 years)

Few injuries occur during the first year of life. As soon as the child learns to move about the incidence of injury increases. This increases further as the child learns to walk and then develops this into running and boisterous play, accounting for the high incidence of oro-dental injury between 2 and 3 years of age (Fig. 1.1). As the child develops, he or she exhibits greater awareness of possible dangers and learns defensive reflex strategies such as 'hands out', and suffers fewer consequences of accidents.

A small but important cause of damage is non-accidental injury (NAI). Approximately half the children abused in this way exhibit facial injuries. Suspicion should be aroused when the history given by the parent does not appear to fit the clinical findings. This topic will be covered in more detail in the section on injuries to the deciduous dentition.

Junior school years (5–11 years)

During this time, accidents in the school playground become common. They are usually falls resulting from play, running wildly, and slipping or colliding with another child. This is also the age at which children start to acquire bicycles, and accidents involving these often result in damage to the teeth. Occasionally, the results are spectacular with damage to many teeth as well as the chin and lips. The fact that many injuries take place before the teeth are fully mature means that special techniques are needed to enable such damaged teeth to develop as far as possible to full maturity.

Secondary school years (11–18 years)

During the teenage years many children are involved in contact sports. Injuries sustained in these sports are often the result of falls, collision with another player, or being hit by a stick or ball used in the game being played. This group of injuries, approximately 3%, is amenable to preventive measures such as mouthguards.

Unfortunately, in our increasingly violent society, fights account for more cases of oro-dental injury. Other activities, such as horse-riding, ice-skating, skiing, gymnastics, and swimming may also result in oro-dental injury, often severe.

Young adults

In the later teenage years, in addition to factors already mentioned, the number of traffic accidents resulting in oro-dental injury increases, although the wearing of seat belts appears to reduce both their number and severity for car occupants.

A factor which is present throughout all age groups is that of any significant disability which predisposes to falls. Toddlers, children, and adolescents with epilepsy, especially when poorly controlled, can suffer repeated oro-dental injuries.

In conclusion, any blow to the mouth from almost any cause may result in soft tissue and dento-alveolar damage. Accurate diagnosis and prompt treatment provide the key to successful management and the best outcome for the young patient.

FURTHER READING

Andreasen, J. O. (1981). *Traumatic injuries of the teeth*, (2nd end). Munksgaard, Copenhagen.

Andreasen, J. O. and Andreasen, F. M. (1994). *Textbook and color atlas of traumatic injuries to the teeth*, (3rd edn). Munksgaard, Copenhagen.

Children's Dental Health in the United Kingdom (1993). Office of Population Censuses and Surveys. Social Survey Division. Her Majesty's Stationery Office.

Ellis, R. G. (1960). *The classification and treatment of injuries of the teeth of children*, (4th edn). Year Book Publishers, Chicago.

Friend, L. A. (1967). Root canal morphology in incisor teeth in the 6–15 year old child. *International Endodontology Journal*, **10**, 35–42.

Sane, J. and Ylipaavalniemi, P. (1988). Dental trauma in contact team sports. *Endodontics and Dental Traumatology*, **4**, 164–9.

2   Investigation of oro-dental injuries

2 Investigation of oro-dental injuries

INTRODUCTION

ORO-DENTAL injury is an emergency—prompt assessment and appropriate treatment are needed to ensure the best outcome.

First contact

Occasionally, the practice may be telephoned by a school secretary, worried parent or friend of a child, who has had an accident resulting in oro-dental injury. This provides an opportunity for specific advice to be given, which may improve the prognosis for the damaged tooth/teeth. For example, if a tooth has been avulsed, the person telephoning may be advised to replace the tooth in its socket. The child should then be brought immediately to the surgery, holding the tooth in place with a handkerchief or paper tissue. In the meantime, the surgery is prepared so that when the child arrives, further treatment may be carried out promptly.

HISTORY, EXAMINATION, DIAGNOSIS, AND TREATMENT PLANNING

All regular clinical care is based on an accurate and careful history, followed by thorough examination and special investigations so that the correct diagnosis is made and the appropriate treatment plan drawn up. The importance of a thorough and systematic history, clinical and radiographic examination cannot be overemphasized as this will ensure that, when planning care for a young patient who has suffered oro-dental trauma, nothing of importance will be overlooked.

HISTORY

Medical

Essential general medical questions, for example, cardiac anomalies (to ensure that the patient is protected), hepatitis B (to ensure that the dental team is protected), and those more specific to the injury, such as loss of consciousness at the time of the accident, are noted. A preprinted medical history sheet (Fig. 2.1) is useful, especially as it reduces the risk of omitting important items. In addition, a question related to tetanus prophylaxis status can be included at the bottom of the sheet. On rare occasions, when evidence of more serious head injury becomes apparent (e.g. drowsiness, double vision, bleeding or leakage of clear fluid from the nose, headache, nausea, or vomiting), the child will have to be referred for more specialist attention before the oro-dental injuries are dealt with. The fact that

Fig. 2.1 A medical history proforma which is completed by the patient, parent, or guardian at the first visit.

MEDICAL HISTORY – CONFIDENTIAL

To be completed by Patient, Parent, or Guardian.

No medical problem or infection will exclude you from receiving essential treatment.

Please note that there is no guarantee that a particular operator will carry out your treatment.

No.		
Name		
D.O.B.		

	YES	NO
Are you in good general health?		

Have you had:–

Heart trouble/murmur, high blood pressure, or rheumatic fever?		
Chest trouble or shortness of breath?		
Jaundice or hepatitis?		
Severe bleeding that needed special treatment?		
Is there a family history of bleeding?		
Any operations or serious illnesses?		
A general anaesthetic?		

ARE YOU suffering or HAVE YOU suffered from:–

Diabetes?		
Asthma, Hay fever or eczema?		
Fainting attacks, blackouts or epilepsy?		
If appropriate: Could you be pregnant?		
Is there any chance that you have become infected with HIV?		
Are you allergic to penicillin or any other drugs?		
Are you taking any medicines, tablets, skin creams, ointments or drugs?		

How much do you smoke per day?... How much do you drink per day?...

FURTHER DETAILS (please add anything of medical importance)

CHECKED BY								
DATE	: :	: :	: :	: :	: :	: :	: :	: :

such complications are infrequent, means that the dentist must maintain a heightened level of vigilance to ensure that such signs and symptoms are not overlooked.

Dental, social, and family history

The child's dental experience will be a useful guide to their ability to co-operate when treatment is carried out. As with the medical history, a preprinted sheet is useful (Fig. 2.2). A social and family history will give information as to the parent's attitude to future treatment—especially important when regular visits would be necessary as with, for example, endodontic therapy.

Trauma history

There are six specific questions:

1. When did the injury take place?
2. Where did the injury take place?
3. How did the injury take place?
4. Has treatment been provided elsewhere?
5. Has there been previous trauma?
6. Have all tooth fragments or avulsed teeth been accounted for?

The answers to these questions enable the full implications of all events related to the injury to be assessed.

1. The time interval will indicate, for example, the feasibility of replacing an avulsed tooth in its socket or direct capping for an exposed dental pulp.
2. The site of injury (e.g. a school playing field) will indicate the need for tetanus prophylaxis.
3. The way in which the injury took place may, for example, indicate the need for a change in drug regimen or a head harness in a patient with severe epilepsy to protect them from further falls. If the injury is the result of an accident or an assault, legal action may ensue and it is particularly important that full records are made.
4. Treatment elsewhere, since the accident, may mask the full extent of the injury or make accurate diagnosis difficult—it may, for example, be unclear if a pulp has been exposed or not if a coronal fracture has been restored.
5. A history of previous trauma may explain clinical and/or radiographic findings which may not be consistent with the trauma history (e.g. a calcified root canal apparent immediately after an episode of trauma).
6. If all tooth fragments or teeth cannot be accounted for, it may be necessary to arrange for a chest X-ray to exclude the possibility of inhalation.

EXAMINATION

A thorough and detailed examination of the face, jaws, teeth, and soft tissues is now carried out, together with any special tests and investigations, so that the extent of the injuries may be established and a full diagnosis made. A simple, systematic scheme should be used. Preprinted proformas (Figs 2.2, 2.3, 2.4) are a useful aid and provide a permanent record.

Fig. 2.2   A clinical history and examination proforma (first side) suitable for all young patients.

PAEDIATRIC DENTISTRY	No.
	SURNAME
	First Name

Date of Attendance in Dental Department	d.o.b.	Age

Reason for Attendance	
History of Present Condition	
Dental History	
Medical History	See Front Sheet
Social and Family History	
Dietary History	
Oral Hygiene Habits	
Extra Oral Examination	
Intra Oral Examination	

Continue Overleaf

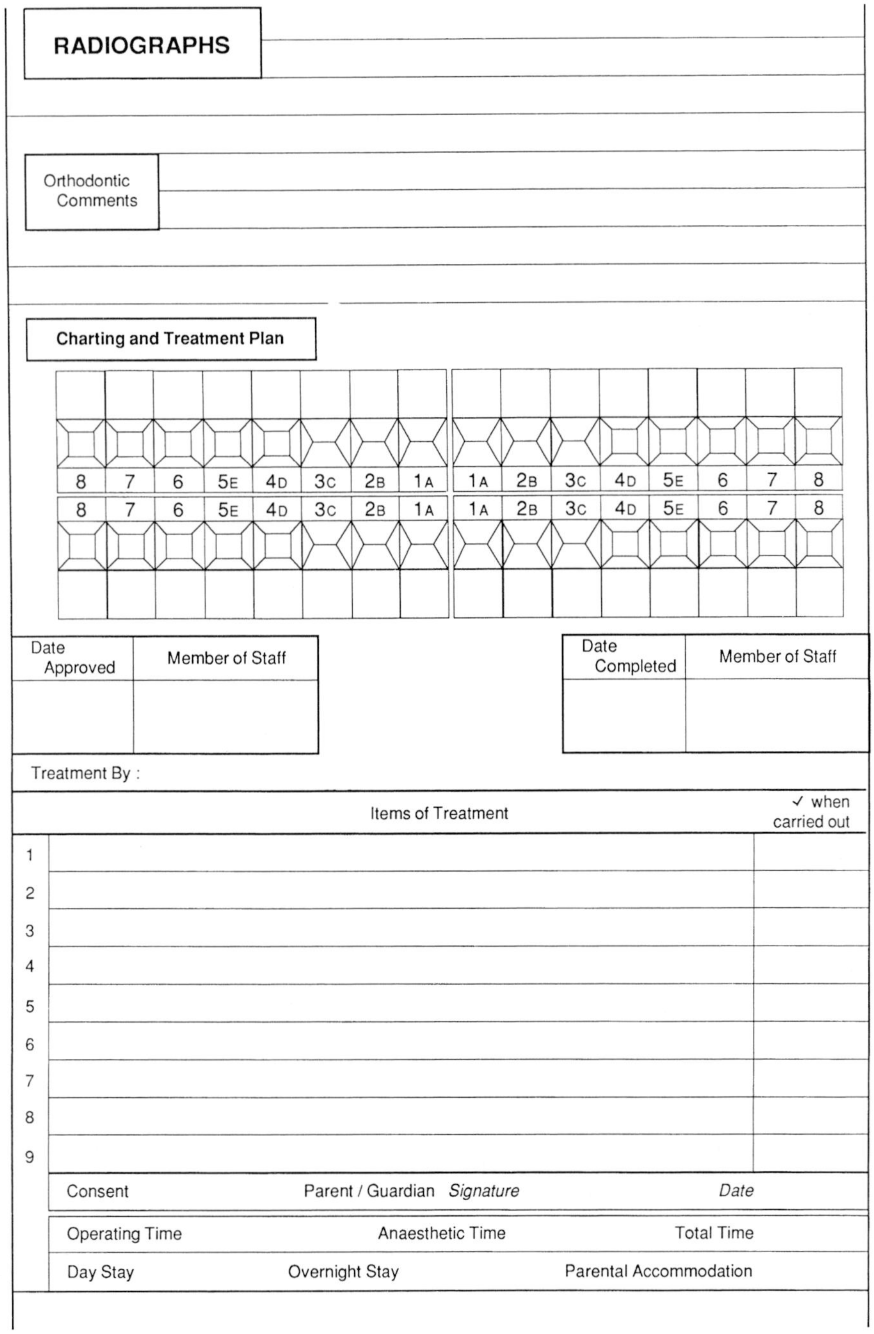

RADIOGRAPHS

Orthodontic Comments

Charting and Treatment Plan

8	7	6	5E	4D	3C	2B	1A	1A	2B	3C	4D	5E	6	7	8
8	7	6	5E	4D	3C	2B	1A	1A	2B	3C	4D	5E	6	7	8

Date Approved	Member of Staff	Date Completed	Member of Staff

Treatment By :

	Items of Treatment	✓ when carried out
1		
2		
3		
4		
5		
6		
7		
8		
9		

Consent	Parent / Guardian *Signature*	*Date*

Operating Time	Anaesthetic Time	Total Time
Day Stay	Overnight Stay	Parental Accommodation

Fig. 2.3 Reverse of history and examination proforma illustrated in Fig. 2.2.

Fig. 2.4 A specific trauma record proforma. The extent and position of crown and/or root fractures may be recorded on the tooth outline, together with other information, provide a permanent record of the injury.

DEPARTMENT OF ORTHODONTICS AND PAEDIATRIC DENTISTRY	No.
INJURED ANTERIOR TEETH	Name.
	First name.

N.B. One tooth or injury per form: enter data in ALL fields (enter data indicated or **Y** for **yes**, **N** for **no**)

Root: Immature? Mature? *(please circle)*

DRAW THE EXTENT OF INJURY

FDI Code for Tooth (two digits) [ ]

Trauma Classification (two digits) [ ]

Trauma Number ....

Today's date ..../...................../.................

Original trauma number..................

Date of Accident ..../...................../.................

Data Interval (yrs) ....

When? [Hours & Minutes] ....
(if appropriate)

Where? ....
(playground, home, road, other)

How? ....
(fall, bicycle, car, fight, sport)

Relevant medical history? ....
(enter yes or no)

Radiographs?   USO .... IOP .... OPG .... Other ....
*(enter yes or no as appropriate **or** specify)*

Vitality tests: Ethyl Chloride .... Electric Pulp Tester .... LD ....

                Hot Gutta Percha .... Test Cavity ....
                (enter +ve, -ve or 'not done' as appropriate or EPT reading)

Malocclusion: ....   Size of Overjet (mm) ....

Displacement ....   Direction e.g. M,L,D,P,I,E .... Amount (mm) ....

Interference with Occlusion? ....   Tender to percussion? ....

Mobility *(grade)* ....   Colour of tooth? .... *(normal, grey, pink, red)*

Draining sinus? ....   Ankylosis? ....

Labial tenderness? ....   Labial swelling? ....

Other injuries?   (head) ....   (jaw) ....   (other) ....

If yes, describe treatment ....

Emergency treatment before arriving .... Specify ....

Systemic antibiotic therapy? ....   If so specify ....

Tetanus prophylaxis? ....   Dental treatment carried out today *(specify)*.....................

....

Arrangements for follow up *(enter details)* ....

Extra-oral examination

A general appraisal of the patient should be made and any cuts, abrasions, swelling, or bruises noted. A simple line drawing can be made in the notes to indicate the extent of the injuries. The bony borders of the maxilla and mandible should be palpated, unless the extent of any oedema makes this too uncomfortable. In addition, the temporo-mandibular joint should be palpated during opening and closing of the mouth. Deviation on opening and closing may indicate a fracture of the neck of the condyle on one side. Extra-oral wounds, particularly of the lips, should be palpated gently to detect the presence of any tooth fragments or foreign bodies.

Intra-oral examination

The oral soft tissues and gingivae are examined for bruises, abrasions, or cuts, general health, and a careful record made.

The state of occlusal development should be examined, and any occlusal problems, especially related to the trauma, noted. A full orthodontic assessment, taking into account any specific problems with individual traumatized teeth can be made at a later date. This avoids hasty, and often inappropriate, decisions being made at a time when the child and parents are in an emotional state.

A full dental charting is carried out so that any other relevant problems, such as dental caries, are not overlooked.

The traumatized teeth may now be examined more closely. A note is made of the extent of any coronal injury from slight crazing of the enamel to complex coronal fractures involving enamel, dentine, pulp and (sometimes) cementum. The position of the tooth/teeth should be noted as should any abnormal mobility, tenderness, or displacement. It is often useful to draw the extent of any dental injury on the trauma record proforma (Fig. 2.4). If teeth have been displaced, it should now be determined if there is interference with the opposing teeth, preventing proper closure. Tenderness of a tooth or group of teeth is suggestive of displacement or alveolar fracture.

Special investigations

Assessment of vitality

Teeth which have recently been injured, frequently fail to respond to conventional vitality testing. Also, the patient may be so distressed following their accident, that it is impossible to obtain a reliable interpretation of any stimulus applied to the teeth—for example, the slight pressure from an electric pulp tester probe, placed on a tooth which is tender to palpation, may be misinterpreted as a positive response to electrical stimulation. Nevertheless, it is important to attempt to obtain a response to such testing to provide a baseline for the interpretation of future results and to assist in assessing the prognosis for maintenance of tooth vitality in the long term.

Several methods for assessing pulp vitality have been described. For general clinical purposes, thermal and electrical stimulation of teeth is satisfactory. However, teeth tested soon after trauma may be concussed and fail to respond. It can be several months before the ability of the tooth to respond returns; decisions with regard to loss of vitality may, therefore, have to be delayed for a considerable period. Apparently undamaged adjacent teeth are often used as a 'control', but the fact that these teeth may also have been injured should not be overlooked.

Thermal vitality testing

Ethyl chloride is usually used for this test—a cotton pledget or roll is soaked with ethyl chloride, evaporation allowed for some seconds and the resulting very cold cotton wool applied to the labial surface of the tooth (Fig. 2.5). It is a simple, cheap method, but the intensity of the stimulus is not controlled and may, therefore, be difficult to reproduce.

Hot gutta percha has also been used—a stick of gutta percha is softened in a hot air heater and then applied to the middle of the labial surface of the tooth to be tested (Fig. 2.6). It is important to coat the tooth surface first with petroleum jelly (Vaseline) to prevent the gutta percha from sticking to the tooth and causing pain. Despite difficulties in standardizing this test, it does provide a reasonably reliable result even in teeth with immature root form.

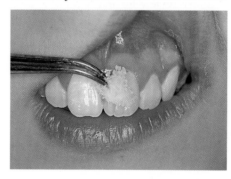 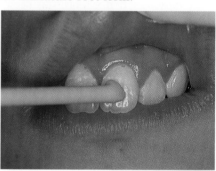

Fig. 2.5 Thermal stimulation (cold) of 21 with a cotton wool pellet soaked with ethyl chloride. As this intense cold can elicit a painful response, there should be only the briefest initial contact. The contact time may then be increased as necessary.

Fig. 2.6 Thermal stimulation (hot) of 21 with hot gutta percha. Again, there should only be the briefest initial contact. The tooth should be coated with a thin film of petroleum jelly to prevent the gutta percha from sticking to the enamel.

Electrical vitality testing

A variety of electrical devices have been developed for testing pulp vitality. One design which has been found to give consistent and reliable results is the Analytic Technology pulp tester (Fig. 2.7). The instrument delivers an electric current in a continuous series of 10 millisecond pulses with the stimulus level indicated by a digital read-out with a scale range of 0–80. The tooth is dried, the conducting tip of the tester is coated with a suitable electrolyte (e.g. acidulated phosphate fluoride gel) and placed against the tooth. When rubber gloves are worn by the clinician an additional electrode is held by the patient to ensure completion of the electrical circuit. Integrity of the circuit is confirmed by illumination of an LED near the tip of the probe (Fig. 2.8). The intensity of the stimulus increases automatically with time, the rate of increase being preset by the dentist. When the patient indicates that they can feel the stimulus, the probe is lifted from the tooth. The digital read-out remains for 10 seconds. When the probe is applied to another tooth the instrument resets itself. In clinical practice, this electric pulp tester is simple to use, with the advantage that readings taken over several visits can be compared.

Nevertheless, no pulp testing method is completely reliable. A poor correlation has been shown between the histological condition of the pulp and vitality test results, to the extent that teeth with necrotic pulps have been known to respond to electric pulp testers. The interpretation of such results is further complicated by the fact that injured teeth, especially involving luxation, frequently show a reduced or negative response. Also, teeth with an immature root anatomy (i.e. most oro-dental injuries in children) often show little or no response whether

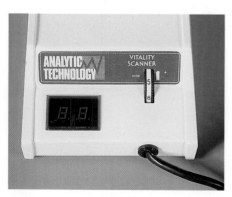

Fig. 2.7 Analytic Technology electric pulp tester with digital read-out.

or not they have been injured. On the other hand, teeth undergoing orthodontic movement often show a heightened response. To improve the reliability of such tests, two methods (one thermal and one electrical) are often used.

Another, non-invasive, method which is undergoing clinical development at the time of writing, is *laser Doppler flowmetry*, a method which attempts to identify the presence or absence of the flow of blood through the tooth. This will clearly be of great benefit in all types of assessment, but most particularly in cases where the blood flow and innervation of the tooth has been interrupted (e.g. replanted teeth) and stimulation of the nerve cannot be expected to be successful for many weeks because of the slowness of re-innervation. One other method is the *test cavity*. This is probably the most reliable method but more difficult to justify as, unlike the other methods, it is invasive. One justification for its use may be when a tooth has been kept under review for many months and the results of vitality testing and radiographic examination continue to be equivocal. In such circumstances, a test cavity will enable a firm diagnosis to be made and appropriate treatment carried out.

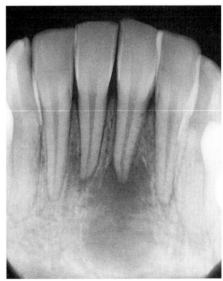

Fig. 2.8 Electric pulp tester probe on tooth; illumination of the LED confirms the integrity of the electrical circuit.

RADIOGRAPHIC EXAMINATION

The use of extra-oral and intra-oral radiographs are indispensable in the diagnosis of oro-dental trauma.

Extra-oral views

The two main views used are the panoramic tomograph and lateral soft tissue view, using an occlusal (57 mm × 76 mm) film.

Panoramic tomograph

This well-established view provides a survey of the whole of the maxilla and mandible including parts of the zygomatic arches and both mandibular condyles. Fractures in the body of the mandible and the alveolus are easily visualized. Although the posterior teeth are well shown, a disadvantage of the technique is that the front of the mouth is usually unclear or distorted due to superimposition of the spinal column (Fig. 2.9). An example of this may be seen in Fig. 2.10

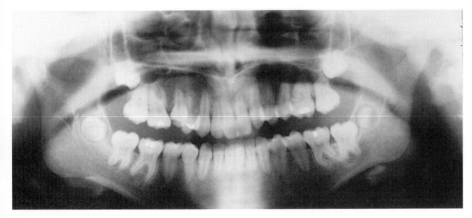

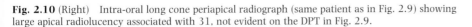

Fig. 2.9 Dental panoramic tomograph (DPT) showing all the teeth but with poor resolution near the midline.

Fig. 2.10 (Right)   Intra-oral long cone periapical radiograph (same patient as in Fig. 2.9) showing large apical radiolucency associated with 31, not evident on the DPT in Fig. 2.9.

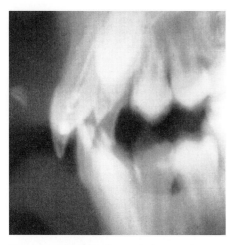

Fig. 2.11 Lateral radiograph showing foreign body in the upper lip.

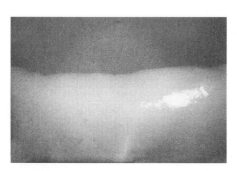

Fig. 2.12 Radiograph showing foreign bodies/debris in the lower lip. The X-ray film is placed in the labial sulcus, between the lip and the teeth, and exposed for approximately half the normal time.

where the lower left central incisor, which had suffered lateral luxation a year before and failed to respond to vitality tests, has a large periapical radiolucency visible on an intra-oral film but not on the panoramic tomograph.

Lateral soft tissue view

This view is taken by reducing the exposure by between one-half and two-thirds. An occlusal size film is used for lateral views or an intra-oral size film for an anterior view of the lip. Any foreign body, such as a tooth fragment, will be clearly visible (Figs 2.11, Fig 2.12).

Intra-oral views

The two intra-oral views used in the assessment of the effects of trauma are the periapical and the standard occlusal.

Periapical radiography

This is the most common view—it is easy to carry out and provides excellent resolution of the tooth and surrounding structures. Two methods are in current use —the paralleling technique and the bisecting angle technique.

The *paralleling view* is recommended as it provides an accurate image with minimal distortion. The film is placed in the mouth at right angles to the plane of the tooth using a special film holder. This enables the film and long axis of the tooth to be parallel to each other, ensuring that the central ray of the X-ray beam is at right angles to the tooth and film (Fig. 2.13). It is easy and quick to use and as views taken in this way are reproducible, more confidence may be placed in interpreting changes from one film to the next.

The *bisecting angle technique* is widely used and has the apparent advantage that additional special equipment is not needed. However, it is much more prone to error and as the views are not reproducible, great caution must be exercised when interpreting follow-up films. Occasionally, as in small mouths, where there is

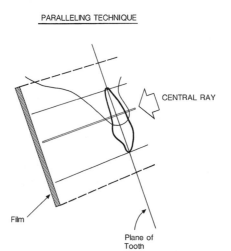

Fig. 2.13 Schematic representation of the relationship between the X-ray film and tooth in the 'paralleling technique'.

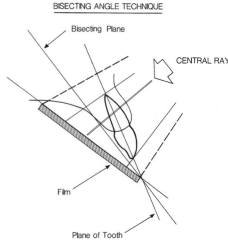

Fig. 2.14 Schematic representation of the relationship between the X-ray film and tooth in the 'bisecting angle technique'.

limitation of opening or the mouth is especially sore as a result of injury, it is necessary to use the technique instead of the paralleling technique. In this technique, when the film is placed in the mouth, an angle is formed between the plane of the film and the long axis of the tooth. The line which bisects this angle is estimated in the mind's eye and the central ray of the X-ray beam directed at right angles to this line (Fig. 2.14). This technique is also easy to use but much more prone to distortion, especially in the apical region and, as has already been mentioned, does not provide reproducible views. A well-taken periapical film provides the dentist with an excellent view of the tooth and its surrounding tissues (Fig. 2.15).

Occlusal radiography

Occlusal views may be taken of both upper and lower anterior teeth. The film may be placed widthways (long axis orientated from left to right) or lengthways (long axis orientated antero-posteriorly) and the tube angled at approximately 70° to the vertical. This view shows lateral or extrusive luxation more reliably than periapical views and when used in conjunction with a periapical view will ensure that root fractures are not overlooked (see also Chapter 5 on root fractures).

For the very young child, who may have difficulty in co-operating sufficiently, the mother can assist by holding the film in place while supporting the child on her lap.

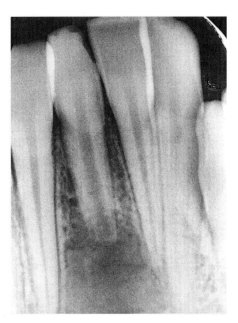

Fig. 2.15 Example of intra-oral long cone periapical radiograph showing 41 and the associated tissues.

FURTHER READING

Andreasen, J. O. and Andreasen, F. M. (1994). Examination and diagnosis of dental injuries. *Textbook and color atlas of traumatic injuries to the teeth*, (3rd edn), Chapter 5. Munksgaard, Copenhagen.

Kopel, H. M. and Johnson, R. (1985). Examination and assessment of children with orodental trauma. *Endodontics and Dental Traumatology*, **1**, 155–9.

3 Injuries affecting the deciduous dentition

3 Injuries affecting the deciduous dentition

INTRODUCTION

MOST injuries to the deciduous dentition take place between the ages of 1 and 3 years (See Fig. 1.1) when children are first learning to walk, and then, later, to run, climb, and play adventurously. The thinner and more elastic alveolar bone found in these young children means that teeth are more likely to be displaced, with associated fracture of the alveolar plate, than suffer crown or root fracture. In older children (4–6 years), physiological resorption, which reduces the root length, also predisposes to displacement or avulsion. The more vertical position of the teeth may also be a factor in the greater proportion of displacement injuries seen in this age group.

The effect of injury in the deciduous dentition falls into three categories:

(1) immediate damage to the teeth and/or oral tissues;
(2) sequelae of damage to the oral tissues often first seen by the dentist when the patient presents 'late'; and
(3) indirect effects of trauma to the permanent dentition caused by damage to the deciduous teeth—only apparent once the permanent teeth have erupted or, perhaps, should have erupted.

EPIDEMIOLOGY

As with the general section on epidemiology, the limitations of the way in which epidemiological data is obtained must be borne in mind. One such study showed that the most common injury found on routine examination was fracture of enamel, comprising 15% of a child population aged 5 years or less. The overall pattern of injury was clearly different from that of permanent teeth (Table 3.1; cf. Table 1.1).

CLASSIFICATION

Injury to the deciduous dentition is classified in the same way as the permanent dentition (Chapter 1), although the distinction between concussion and sub-luxation is probably inappropriate. The pattern of injury, however, appears to be different, presumably because of fundamental differences in the nature of the trauma causing the injury and the greater resilience of the tissues involved in this age group.

Table 3.1 Epidemiology of perceived damage to deciduous teeth: A total of 313 (21%) teeth in 1509 children

Type of injury	Percentage of total number of injured teeth %
Fracture of enamel	73
Fracture involving enamel and dentine	10
Fracture involving enamel, dentine, and pulp	0.3
Displacement or mobility (no fracture of crown)	0.3
Displacement or mobility (with fracture of enamel)	1.3
Displacement or mobility (with fracture of enamel and dentine)	1.1
Displacement or mobility (with fracture into pulp)	0
Discoloration (no other sign of fracture)	5
Tooth loss due to trauma	9
Total	100

After Cleaton-Jones *et al.* unpublished data.

AETIOLOGY

Injury during the first year of life is unusual but may result from the child being dropped, or falling from its pram. Once the child starts to walk the number of falls increases, and continues to increase as the child starts to run, reflected in the increased number of injuries between 1 and 3 years of age (see Fig. 1.1).

Abrasions and lacerations of the oral and perioral tissues are a common feature of injury in this age group.

Non-accidental injury (NAI)

A small number of children are victims of deliberate and, sometimes, systematic injury by their parent(s), or other adults involved in their care. Although oro-dental injuries are rarely the presenting problem, from time to time the child's first contact with a health care professional may be with the dentist. Approximately 50% of non-accidental injuries are to the face. For this reason all dentists caring for children should be aware of the possibility of non-accidental injury.

Physical abuse can be defined as any injury where there is definite knowledge or reasonable suspicion that the injury was inflicted, or knowingly not prevented, by any person having custody, charge, or care of the child.

Suspicion may be aroused by an apparent discrepancy in the trauma history provided by the parent(s) and the injuries found on examination. Also, the parents may each give a different version of the trauma history. A torn upper labial frenum is an unusual injury and is sometimes due to NAI (Fig. 3.1). The injury results from contact with the back of the hand as it sweeps upwards and across the mouth, the adult lashing out especially when the child is crying persistently. Further causes for concern are the presence of injuries which appear to be of different ages and a child who attends repeatedly with injuries to the mouth and teeth.

Since 1980, there has been increasing awareness of the extent of child abuse. As a result, organizations with responsibility for child care have established effective protocols for the appropriate response to reports of any form of child abuse. In the United Kingdom, each local authority has a Child Protection Register and the officer responsible for this can be contacted 24 hours of the day

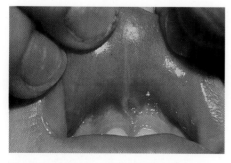

Fig. 3.1 Torn upper labial frenum in a 4-year-old child possibly associated with non-accidental injury (NAI) (by courtesy of Dr C. J. Hobbs).

and night. In case of difficulty, help can also be obtained from the local police, National Society for the Prevention of Cruelty to Children, or Child Line. It is important to arrange an appointment to review the oro-dental injury as this provides a suitable opportunity to check that the correct action has been taken in regard to the suspected non-accidental injury.

SPECIAL CONSIDERATIONS

Injuries to the oro-dental structures of young children evoke a strong, sometimes hysterical, reaction from the parent(s). It is especially important for the dentist to remain calm and reassuring. This helps the parent(s) to relax and be more able to accept the treatment proposed by the dentist. This can be particularly important when no active intervention is deemed necessary. Parents can find it difficult to understand that the best management is often allowing damaged tissues time to heal and then reviewing the situation later.

EXAMINATION

Young children, particularly when they have sustained an injury, are often difficult to examine. The history, which has to be taken from the parent, is sometimes of only limited value as the accident which caused the injury was not witnessed.

When examining the child it is often necessary to exercise mild restraint to ensure that a thorough examination is carried out. This can be done by seating the parent on a chair opposite the dentist with the child sitting on the parent's lap, but facing away from the dentist. The child can then be gently lowered backwards so that its head is on the dentist's knees or lap (Fig. 3.2). The parent can now hold the child and, if necessary, restrain his or her hands and feet. If the dentist holds the side of the head with the ball of the hand, side-to-side movements are also reduced. The dentist can now carry out a thorough examination including the usual dental charting. When it is clear that successful treatment will only be possible under general anaesthesia, further, detailed examination may be delayed. It is important to explain to the parent(s) the intention to carry out further examination under general anaesthesia (EUA) and carry out the appropriate treatment at the same time. The parent(s) need to be made aware of the implications of this course of action before being asked to sign the consent form. For example, it may be found necessary to extract more teeth than at first seemed likely—the parent(s) need to be prepared for this eventuality.

Radiographs should, ideally, be obtained although this is often difficult in the young child, especially following an accident. The child's co-operation can sometimes be gained by the parent holding the X-ray film in the child's mouth (Fig. 3.3). With a small child, a 'periapical' size film (21 mm × 34 mm), held transversely, may be used to obtain an occlusal view.

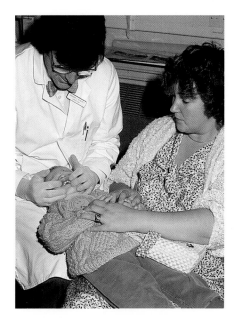

Fig. 3.2 Intra-oral examination of the young child with head on operator's lap and the parent controlling the child's arms.

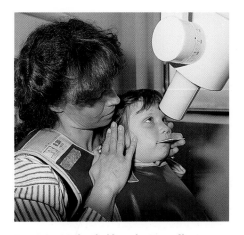

Fig. 3.3 Mother holding the X-ray film in a very young child.

TREATMENT

Many oro-dental injuries in the deciduous dentition will require little more than reassurance, time to allow the damaged tissues to heal followed by regular monitoring (usually at the time of routine recall visits) to ensure that no adverse sequelae are developing.

Nevertheless, there are times when active intervention will be necessary and the principles laid down elsewhere in this book for the care of permanent teeth may be used as the basis for the management of injury in the deciduous dentition, albeit with some clear differences.

As the greater proportion of injuries in the deciduous dentition involve very young children, their ability to cope with treatment is often a limiting factor, even with inhalation sedation. If treatment is to be arranged under general anaesthesia, a fairly radical approach may have to be adopted to avoid a repeat anaesthetic within a short time. Under such circumstances, teeth with an uncertain prognosis would be extracted rather than subjected to heroic restorative techniques.

1. Crown fractures

(a) enamel
(b) enamel + dentine
(c) enamel + dentine + pulp
(d) enamel + dentine + cementum +/– pulp

In (a) and (b) it is usually sufficient to carry out some simple smoothing of rough enamel. If the fracture in (b) is extensive, and the child co-operative, the tooth can be restored with etch-retained composite. When the fracture results in pulp exposure (c), a formocresol pulpotomy can be carried out in a co-operative child, otherwise the tooth is extracted. In (d) the extent of the damage usually leaves little choice but extraction of the tooth.

2. Root fractures

If the root fracture results in excessive mobility of the coronal fragment, extraction is again the treatment of choice. Where the fracture line is nearer the apex, or the tooth is only moderately mobile it may be left to heal, which is usually by interposition of connective tissue between the fragments. If the coronal fragment subsequently becomes non-vital, it should be extracted and the apical portion left to resorb physiologically.

3. Luxation injuries

(a) concussion
(b) subluxation (loosening)
(c) intrusive luxation (intrusion)
(d) extrusive luxation (extrusion)
(e) lateral luxation
(f) total luxation (avulsion)

(a) and (b) because of difficulties with diagnosis in the very young child, it is probably sensible to consider concussion and subluxation as a single entity. Management of these injuries, once clinical and radiographic examination have excluded other injury, is almost invariably that of reassurance and regular review.

(c) intrusion in this age group can be severe. Sometimes the clinical appearance is that of avulsion; only when radiographs are taken are the teeth revealed, displaced a considerable distance apically. Nevertheless, in almost all instances of intrusion, reassurance and observation are all that is required. Most intruded deciduous teeth will re-erupt over a period of a few months. Only if there is clear evidence that the intruded tooth is in contact with the underlying successional tooth should consideration be given to removing the intruded tooth. A relatively unusual complication is infection, in which case the intruded tooth/teeth should be extracted.

(d) extruded deciduous teeth are usually extracted. Repositioning such teeth may result in damage to underlying permanent teeth. In addition, providing an adequate splint to support the repositioned tooth may be difficult in a very young child.

(e) lateral luxation will often need no active intervention. If the tooth has been displaced labially, lip pressure will frequently result in natural realignment over the next two to three weeks. Similarly, a palatal displacement will tend to be repositioned naturally by tongue pressure, over about a week. If the displaced tooth is interfering with the occlusion, the child postures the mandible forward to avoid the premature contact and as the tooth moves forward, continues to increase this posturing until the tooth is far enough labially for the lower teeth to occlude palatally again, at which time the posturing is no longer needed.

(f) avulsed deciduous teeth are not usually replanted because of the possibility of interfering with the underlying successional tooth. Parents are often upset by this initially but usually find the explanation acceptable.

Among the complications that can arise following these injuries are:

(i)   darkening of the tooth, which can lighten again, especially if the initial colour change takes place quite quickly after injury

(ii) calcification of the pulp chamber and root canal, which results in a yellow discoloration of the crown

(iii) loss of pulp vitality with chronic apical infection and the development of a buccal sinus. If this is not treated, normal, physiological resorption may be disrupted.

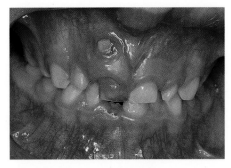

Fig. 3.4 Apex of chronically infected, non-vital 51 being deflected labially by erupting permanent successor (11).

The permanent successor may be deflected or may push the deciduous tooth out of the way, the apex of the deciduous tooth perforating the buccal plate and overlying mucosa (Fig. 3.4). The deciduous tooth should be extracted in such cases, to allow the permanent tooth to erupt unhindered.

LATE PRESENTATION

Undoubtedly, many deciduous tooth injuries go unnoticed, or are untreated at the time of injury because the parents consider the injury to be trivial and, therefore, see no reason to consult the dentist. Occasionally, the results of injury are noticed by the dentist clinically or following radiographic examination. Root fractures are sometimes 'found' when radiographs have been taken for another purpose.

A common presentation is darkening of the tooth. When a problem supervenes, the usual careful clinical and radiographic assessment is carried out and a suitable plan of treatment devised. This must be discussed fully with the parents —they are often reluctant, for example, to agree to the loss of discoloured teeth that are apparently causing the child no problem. However, in this child with discoloured teeth, although the clinical appearance of the buccal mucosa is normal (Fig. 3.5), a radiograph of the region shows a large apical radiolucency

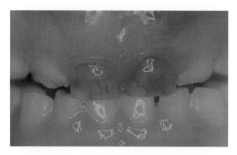

Fig. 3.5 Discoloured 51, 61 with healthy buccal mucosa.

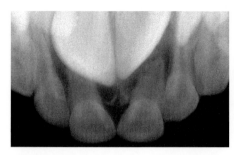

Fig. 3.6 Radiograph of 51, 61 from patient in Fig. 3.5, showing chronic apical infection with bone loss.

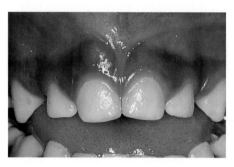

Fig. 3.7 Symptomless 51 with small buccal swelling which the parent had not noticed.

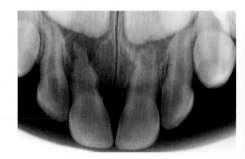

Fig. 3.8 Radiograph of 51, 61 (same patient as in Fig. 3.7), showing infection and root resorption affecting 51.

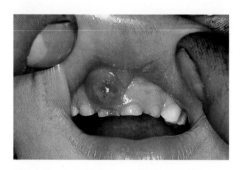

Fig. 3.9 Acute infection affecting 51 following pulp necrosis resulting from trauma some months previously.

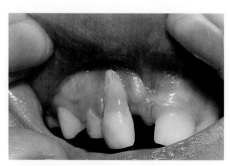

Fig. 3.10 Lateral luxation of 51: late presentation with tooth retained by palatal soft tissue only.

on each upper central deciduous incisor (Fig. 3.6). This case also serves to illustrate the importance of obtaining radiographs for such patients.

In the case illustrated in Figs 3.7 and 3.8 there were no symptoms but the mother felt that the tooth was unsightly and wanted treatment to improve the appearance. The parents had not noticed the 'gum boil' labially. Radiographic examination revealed partially resorbed roots, apical radiolucency associated with 51 due to chronic infection, and loss of definition of the root canal, probably resulting from internal resorption before the pulp became non-vital. The prudent treatment was to extract the tooth before acute infection developed and to reduce the risk of damage to the permanent successor.

Commonly, non-vital teeth have to be extracted, but from time to time (often as the result of parental pressure!) non-vital pulp therapy may be used to avoid extraction. The success rate for this form of treatment is not high and the potential for residual infection causing damage to the permanent successor should not be overlooked.

Sometimes, acute signs and symptoms develop requiring urgent extraction of the infected teeth (Fig. 3.9). Unlike the considerable facial and/or submandibular swelling that can arise from dento-alveolar abscesses affecting deciduous molars, soft tissue swelling caused by deciduous incisors rarely involves more than a relatively small amount of tissue, because of the thin labial plate of bone and proximity of the root apices to the alveolar mucosa. Occasionally, with lateral luxation involving the labial plate the bone and soft tissues heal leaving a moribund deciduous incisor hanging on by minimal soft tissue attachment (Fig. 3.10).

When assessing young children who have suffered oro-dental injury the possibility of previous trauma should always be borne in mind, especially when there are unexpected clinical and/or radiographic findings.

DAMAGE TO SUCCESSIONAL TEETH

The proximity of the root of the deciduous incisor to the crown of its permanent successor during early childhood (Figs 3.11, 3.12) means that when a deciduous tooth is injured there is significant potential for damage to the permanent successor. The effect may be either:

Direct: for example, when the root apex of an intruded deciduous central incisor impinges on the labial surface of the developing permanent incisor; or

Indirect: for example, when a deciduous tooth becomes non-vital, periapical infection can damage the immature labial enamel of the underlying permanent tooth.

When small children present with injury in the deciduous dentition the possible effect on the developing permanent teeth is often one of their parents' first concerns. In many cases, our ability to limit damage by some form of intervention is small, as damage to the permanent tooth often takes place at the time of injury and treatment will influence the outcome of the injury to only a minor extent.

From the study of Andreasen and Ravn (1971), the most important factor in determining whether damage to the successional tooth will result or not, seems to be the age of the child, the highest incidence of damage to permanent successors following injury to the deciduous teeth taking place between 0 and 2 years of age (Table 3.2). Table 3.2 also suggests that the probability of a young child under 4 years of age having damage to permanent teeth is of the order of 60%. Nevertheless, accurate diagnosis at the time of injury, ensuring that appropriate care is prescribed, combined with careful follow-up so that should pulp necrosis

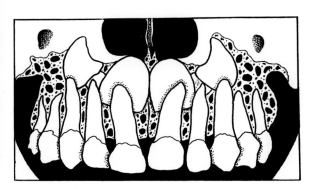

Fig. 3.11 Schematic representation of anterior maxillary region of a young child showing the close relationship of the roots of the deciduous teeth to their permanent successors.

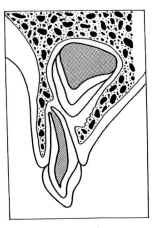

Fig. 3.12 Schematic representation of the incisor region of a young child showing the labio-lingual and vertical relationships of the root of the upper deciduous incisor and its permanent successor.

Table 3.2 Association of age of patient and subsequent damage to permanent successors

Age (yrs)	Total	No defect	Damage	%
0–2	62	23	39	63
3–4	43	20	23	53
5–6	88	67	21	24
7–9	20	15	5	25

After Andreasen and Ravn (1971).

and apical infection supervene, effective treatment may be instituted promptly, will in many cases prevent hypoplasia or hypomineralization affecting the permanent successors.

The most serious deciduous tooth injuries in terms of damage to the permanent successors are seen to be intrusive luxation, when 69% of injuries resulted in damage to the permanent successor, followed by avulsion (52%), extrusive luxation and subluxation (each 34%) (See Table 3.2). These are injuries which result in superficial damage to, or bodily displacement of, the underlying tooth germs (Table 3.3). Other types of injury do not appear to result in damage to the developing tooth germs. The permanent teeth most often affected are the central incisors. The permanent lateral incisors are much less frequently affected, especially at an early age, because they lie palatal to the developing central incisors and are, therefore, protected. However, if the trauma is severe the lateral incisors can also be damaged.

Table 3.3 Damage of permanent successors by type of injury

Injury Type	Total	No defect	Enamel Defect	%
Subluxation	35	23	12	34
Extrusion	76	50	26	34
Intrusion	36	11	25	69
Avulsion	27	13	14	52

After Andreasen and Ravn (1971).

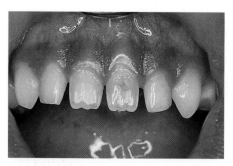

Fig. 3.13 Yellow-brown discoloration affecting 41 but not, apparently, 31 following injury to the deciduous predecessors.

The effect on the successional tooth may be a mild white or yellow-brown discoloration (Fig. 3.13). In this example, the lower right central incisor has a discoloured patch labially and the lower left central appears undamaged. However, an intra-oral radiograph shows that it has not escaped damage—beneath the immature gingiva there is a ring of enamel hypoplasia (Fig. 3.14).

In the older child, resorption of the roots of the deciduous incisors, and the state of development of the permanent incisors, means that injury to the deciduous teeth tends to result in crown or root dilaceration of the permanent teeth. In the case illustrated in Figs 3.15 and 3.16, injury to the deciduous teeth has resulted in dilaceration of the upper left central incisor at the junction of the crown and root (Fig. 3.17). The lateral view shows clearly the malpositioned crown with the the major part of the root properly aligned within the jaw. Some years later, following orthodontic treatment, the crown is properly aligned and the root is now displaced labially. Clinically, the tooth has a satisfactory appearance, although the alveolar mucosa is distorted by the root apex (Figs 3.18, Fig 3.19) In the majority of cases where injury in the deciduous dentition has resulted in damage to the labial enamel of the permanent successor, the problem will be amenable to cosmetic treatment, once the tooth has erupted.

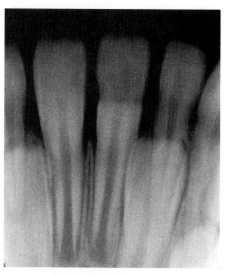

Fig. 3.14 Intra-oral radiograph of the teeth in Fig. 3.13 which shows that 31 was affected—there is a hypoplastic ring below the gingival margin.

FOLLOW-UP

Regular reviews are clearly important following injury in the deciduous dentition, particularly if the sequelae of injury are not to adversely affect the developing permanent teeth. One problem can be that the child's parents may regard the injury as trivial and, therefore, not bring the child for examination or treatment. Subsequent, insidious, infection within the alveolar bone may go unrecognized until the permanent tooth erupts, resulting in late presentation.

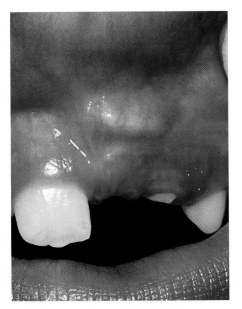

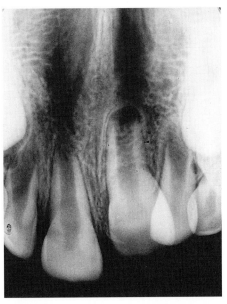

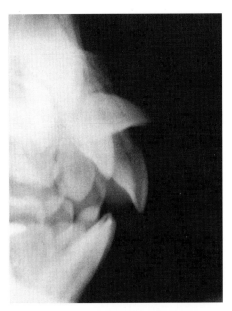

Fig. 3.15 Aberrant eruption of 21 with its incisal edge high in the labial sulcus.

Fig. 3.16 Intra-oral radiograph of the patient in Fig. 3.15 which shows a somewhat distorted root of 21.

Fig. 3.17 Lateral radiograph of the patient in Figs 3.15, 3.16 showing the dilacerate crown of 21, which accounts for its aberrant eruption.

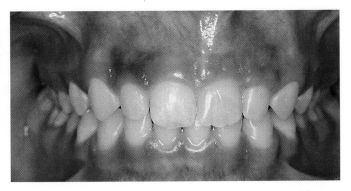

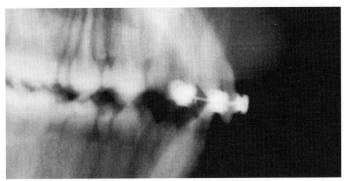

Fig. 3.18 Photograph of the patient shown in Figs 3.15–3.17 following orthodontic treatment which has successfully corrected the angulation of the crown of 21.

Fig. 3.19 Lateral radiograph of the same patient showing the angulation of the root of dilacerate 21 after uprighting its crown.

FURTHER READING

Andreasen, J. O. and Ravn, J. J. (1971) The effect of traumatic injuries to primary teeth on their permanent successors. 2. A clinical and radiographic follow up study of 213 teeth. *Scandinavian Journal* of *Dental Research*, **79**, 284–94.

Andreasen, J. O., Sundström, B., and Ravn J. J. (1971). The effect of traumatic injuries to primary teeth on their permanent successors. 1. A clinical and histologic study of 117 injured permanent teeth. *Scandinavian Journal* of *Dental Research*, **79**, 219–83.

Child Protection (1988). Lambeth, Lewisham and Southwark Area Review Committee.

George, J. E. (1973). Spare the rod: A survey of the battered child syndrome. *Forensic Science*, **2**, 129–67.

Hargreaves, J. A., Cleaton-Jones, P., Roberts G. J., and Leidhal, I. (1985). An epidemiological study of oro-dental trauma in South African children under the age of 5 years. (Unpublished data)

MacIntyre D. R., Jones G. M., and Pinckney R. C. N. (1986). The role of the dental practitioner in the management of non-accidental injury in children. *British Dental Journal*, **161**, 108–10.

Symons A. L., Rowe P. V., and Romaniuk, K. (1987). Dental aspects of child abuse: a review and case reports. *Australian Dental Journal* **32**, 42–7.

4   Crown fracture

4 Crown fracture

CROWN fracture accounts for 75% of fractured teeth and when appropriate treatment is provided the prognosis is good. Coronal damage and fracture are classified according to the tissues involved:

- Fracture of enamel
- Fracture of enamel and dentine
- Fracture of enamel, dentine, and pulp
- Fracture of enamel, dentine, and cementum
- Fracture of enamel, dentine, pulp, and cementum

The impact which causes coronal fracture also results in some degree of luxation injury, usually the milder forms, concussion, and subluxation. As a rule, these additional injuries will not require active treatment. However, when the more severe forms of luxation injury are superimposed on coronal fracture, the management is more complex and the prognosis, inevitably, less certain.

EXAMINATION

Following general assessment of the patient (see Chapter 2) the damaged tooth is examined to determine its colour, translucency, the degree of fracture and any displacement, mobility, and tenderness. It should be remembered that teeth that have recently been subject to injury may be hyper-reactive to manipulation, however gentle. Conventional thermal and electrical vitality testing are then carried out. Although some teeth will not respond at this stage because of the concussive effects of the trauma, useful baseline information is obtained. Indeed, it has been shown that the sooner a tooth develops a response to routine vitality testing after injury, the more likely the long-term survival of the pulp. In cases of persistently equivocal results to clinical and radiographic assessment of tooth vitality, a test cavity may be the only way, at present, of resolving the matter. However, laser Doppler flowmetry may well become an additional tool for assessing pulpal blood flow (and, hence, vitality) but is, as yet, too expensive for general use.

Radiographs are an essential adjunct to clinical examination and assist in the diagnosis and assessment of the extent and severity of additional injuries such as root fracture and luxation.

FRACTURE OF ENAMEL

Enamel fracture, where the coronal fracture is confined to the enamel (Figs 4.1, Fig 4.2), represents approximately 47% of all crown fractures and is the most common dental injury seen in dental practice. The damage may simply be hairline cracks (also described as a separate category—enamel infraction—by some authorities), or may result in loss of enamel. In the absence of other damage, treatment is confined to reassurance and smoothing the roughened enamel

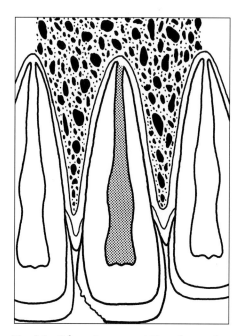

Fig. 4.1 Schematic representation of coronal fracture involving enamel.

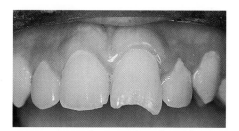

Fig. 4.2 Enamel fracture affecting mesial aspect of 11 and more extensive damage to 21.

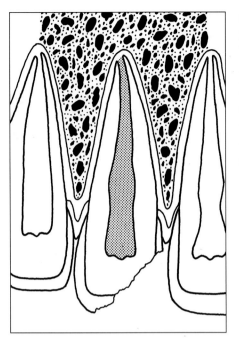

Fig. 4.3 Schematic representation of coronal fracture involving enamel and dentine.

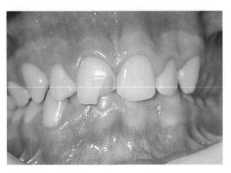

Fig. 4.4 Coronal fracture of 11 involving enamel and dentine.

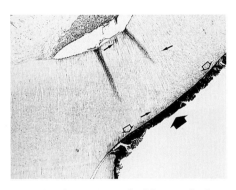

Fig. 4.5 Photomicrograph of demineralized section of a permanent incisor showing plaque accumulation on the fractured dentine surface (large arrow), bacteria entering the dentinal tubules (open arrows), and bacteria migrating towards the pulp (small arrows).

edges. If larger areas of enamel are lost, especially when involving the contact point, the tooth should be restored with etch-retained composite, both for aesthetic reasons and to prevent space loss.

Radiographs

The radiographic findings associated with enamel fracture are usually negative in that they demonstrate the absence of other damage. Nevertheless, they enable the dentist to reassure the patient and the parents as to the limited nature of the injury. The management of root fracture and of luxation injury are considered in Chapters 5 and 6.

FRACTURE OF ENAMEL AND DENTINE

Coronal fracture involving enamel and dentine but without exposure of the dental pulp (Figs 4.3, 4.4) comprises approximately 17% of all tooth fractures. All too often such fractures are left untreated, either because the child and/or parent consider the damage to be trivial and do not seek treatment, or because the dental practitioner believes that the child will not be able to tolerate the clinical procedures involved in restoration. Unfortunately, economic factors may also influence the decision. However, if the exposed dentine is not protected, considerable pulpal irritation can result from direct thermal or chemical stimulation, or from invasion of oral bacteria along the dentinal tubules. Pulp necrosis may then result. In the case illustrated in Fig. 4.5 accumulation of dental plaque on the fractured dentine surface (large arrow) has resulted in bacteria entering the dentinal tubules (open arrows) migrating towards the dental pulp (small arrows) with pulpal inflammation, necrosis, and infection.

Radiographs

Upper anterior occlusal and long cone periapical views of the affected and adjacent teeth should be taken to confirm the extent of the injury, absence of other damage, such as root fracture or luxation injury, and identify any effect resulting from previous injury.

Treatment

Objectives of treatment

(1) to protect the pulp from chemical or thermal insult and bacterial contamination;
(2) to prevent the effects of potentially painful stimuli for the patient;
(3) to prevent tilting of adjacent teeth;
(4) to restore appearance and function.

These objectives may be achieved by covering the exposed dentine with a rapid-setting calcium hydroxide cement (e.g. Dycal). This, in turn, is protected by a suitable restoration, such as an etch-retained composite, which restores both appearance and function (Figs 4.6, 4.7, 4.8).

When a patient is too distressed to tolerate immediate placement of a definitive restoration, the calcium hydroxide cement may be protected in the short term by a layer of etch-retained fissure sealant or by glass ionomer cement and the definitive restoration placed within a few days.

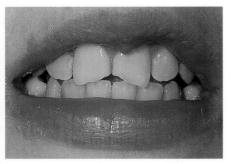

Fig. 4.6 Coronal fracture of 11 and 21 involving enamel and dentine.

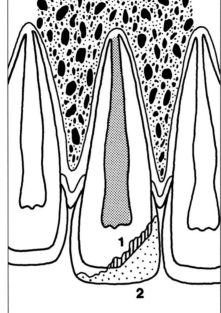

Fig. 4.7 Schematic representation of restoration of coronal fracture involving enamel and dentine: (1) calcium hydroxide cement protecting the dentine surface; (2) etch-retained composite restoration.

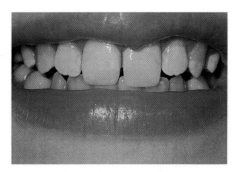

Fig. 4.8 Fractured 11 and 21 (from Fig. 4.6) repaired with etch-retained composite restoration.

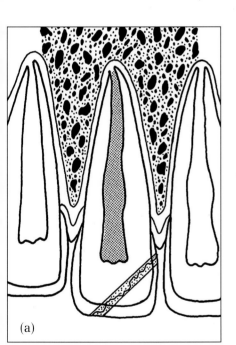

(a)

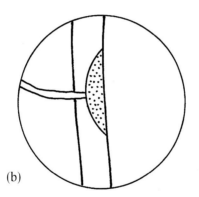

(b)

Fig. 4.9 (a) Schematic representation of broken tooth fragment reattached to tooth with dentine bonding agent. (b) Schematic representation of groove cut in enamel along fracture line and filled with etch-retained composite resin to reinforce reattached fragment in Fig. (a).

If the tooth fragment has been retrieved from the scene of the accident it can sometimes be reattached using a dentine bonding agent and etch-retained composite. Where the dentine overlying the pulp is very thin, secondary or reparative dentine formation is encouraged by placing calcium hydroxide cement over the dentine, held in place with a temporary etch-retained composite restoration. In the meantime, the fragment broken off the tooth is stored in sterile saline. After a month, the composite and the calcium hydroxide are removed and the tooth fragment cemented to the main body of the tooth using a dentine bonding agent. Once the bonding agent has set, the join between the two fragments is reinforced by creating a furrow in the enamel along the fracture line, etching the enamel and restoring the furrow with composite (Fig. 4.9 a, b).

Prognosis

The outcome for teeth with enamel and dentine fracture, particularly with regard to pulp survival, appears to depend mainly on the associated injuries to the supporting tissues and to the stage of root development at the time of injury. Table 4.1 shows that there is a tendency for pulp survival to decrease with increasing tooth maturity. However, this is not the case when the tooth has also suffered intrusive luxation. Intrusive luxation almost invariably results in loss of vitality, irrespective of the state of root maturity. More recent work has shown that 30–40% of intruded immature teeth do not, in fact, become non-vital as had earlier been found.

Although teeth with enamel and dentine fracture rarely become non-vital in the absence of additional injury, there is, nevertheless, some risk of this happening. It is prudent, therefore, to monitor such teeth regularly, which should become part of the patient's regular dental check-ups after the initial phases of care have been completed. It is worth noting that, albeit unusually, teeth can become non-vital six or seven years after the original injury.

Table 4.1 Percentage pulp survival following enamel and dentine fracture in relation to associated periodontal injury

Injury	Immature Teeth %	Mature Teeth %
No luxation	98	96
Concussion	96	90
Subluxation	80	50
Extrusion	60	20
Lateral luxation	70	18
Intrusion	0	0

After Andreasen and Andreasen (1990).

FRACTURE OF ENAMEL, DENTINE, AND PULP

This fracture accounts for approximately 5% of all episodes of trauma and involves enamel and dentine with exposure of the dental pulp (Figs 4.10, 4.11). A successful outcome depends largely on effective management of bacterial contamination at the exposure site. The priority is to treat the exposed pulp as quickly as possible.

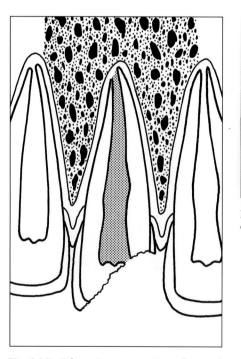

Fig. 4.10 Schematic representation of coronal fracture involving enamel, dentine and pulp.

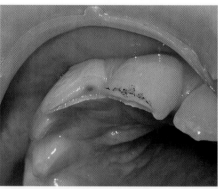

Fig. 4.11 Coronal fracture of 11 involving enamel, dentine, and pulp.

Response of pulp tissue exposed due to trauma

Our understanding of the natural history of pulpal change following traumatic exposure is based on primate studies.

Exposure of the tooth pulp following trauma causes laceration of the pulp at the exposure site and bleeding. Although in contact with the saliva at the exposure site, bacterial colonization of the superficial pulp tissue does not take place immediately. Nevertheless, exposed pulps rarely heal spontaneously and if left untreated, necrosis and infection are almost invariably the outcome.

The immediate result of the tissue damage at the exposure site is haemorrhage, followed by the development of an acute inflammatory reaction in response, initially, to the breakdown products from the damaged tissue and then, probably a little later, to the presence of salivary bacteria. Subsequently, the exposed pulp is covered with a layer of fibrin and blood clot which then becomes colonized by bacteria.

In the first few days after the exposure, tissue changes may be proliferative or destructive. In the former, which the most common reaction, there is pulpal hyperplasia, with herniation of pulp tissue through the breach in the dentine. This response appears to take place irrespective of the size of the exposure. In the latter, there may be abscess formation in the subsurface layers or superficial tissue necrosis.

In these early days following exposure, the inflammation is superficial, extending no more than 2 mm into the pulp beneath. On the few occasions when superficial necrosis takes place, healthy pulp may, nevertheless, be observed 4 mm from the surface. Although the most common response is pulpal hyperplasia, presumably favoured by the regular 'washing' of the exposed pulp surface by saliva, as days go by, impaction of food fragments and debris causes further pulpal damage leading to local abscess formation, persistent inflammation, and, eventually, total pulp necrosis.

It is clear, therefore, that during the first hours and days following the trauma, when the patient usually seeks treatment, the potential for pulp recovery is favourable and a good outcome to treatment designed to maintain pulp health and continued vitality may be expected.

Objectives of treatment

The primary objective of treatment is maintenance of pulp vitality, so that:

1. In immature teeth, root development and maturation may continue.
2. In mature teeth, the adverse consequences of root canal therapy, such as coronal discolouration and brittleness, may be avoided.

Four techniques are available for treating the exposed pulp:

(1) direct pulp capping;
(2) minimal pulpotomy (partial pulpotomy/cornuectomy);
(3) cervical (radical) pulpotomy;
(4) pulpectomy.

There is a lack of consistency in the use of some of these terms. For the sake of clarity, the authors' use of each term will be described at the beginning of the relevant section on treatment. Selection of the appropriate treatment and sequence of clinical procedures depends on an understanding of the biological principles involved and the healing stages which may be expected in teeth treated by these different methods.

Factors affecting therapeutic healing of pulp exposures

The aim of treatment is to maintain a vital pulp, free of inflammation. An understanding of the factors that may influence the outcome of treatment enables the clinician to decide which treatment strategy is appropriate in a given case.

Factors to be considered

Factors which may affect the outcome of healing of an exposed pulp following treatment may be considered under two main headings and a number of subheadings:

1. *Factors associated with the injury*
   (a) size of exposure;
   (b) time since the accident;
   (c) degree of bacterial contamination;
   (d) associated injuries.

2. *Factors associated with treatment*
   (a) presence of a blood clot;
   (b) presence of inflammation;
   (c) operative technique and type of drill used;
   (d) level of pulp amputation;
   (e) choice of pulp medicament.

1. Factors associated with the injury

(a) Size of exposure

There is no evidence to support the statement that fractured teeth with larger exposures have a poorer prognosis. Indeed, in the related field of iatrogenic exposure arising during treatment for caries, no difference in outcome has been shown in relation to the size of the exposure. It has also been shown in traumatically induced pulp exposures, in primates, that the size of the exposure does not affect the ability of the pulp to form a satisfactory calcific barrier beneath calcium hydroxide. Nevertheless, it is possible that the larger the exposure the greater the risk of bacterial contamination and the larger the blood clot on the pulp surface, both factors known to adversely influence healing (see below). However, the idea that the size of the exposure is important is so firmly entrenched that it will be a long time before the prevailing view changes. This is especially difficult to reconcile as the recommended treatment procedures frequently involve surgically increasing the size of the pulp exposure. An explanation for this difference of opinion is that small exposures appear clinically as if only the edge of the pulp is involved. With larger fractures, where the fragment is lost, the pulp associated with the lost fragment remains attached to the main body of the pulp appearing like a pulp polyp protruding from the surface. When seen promptly, before the onset of inflammation, surgical removal of the protruding part of the pulp and placement of calcium hydroxide, could be expected to have a satisfactory outcome.

(b) Time since the accident

The treatment of pulp exposure should be carried out as soon as possible after the accident, preferably within a few hours. The longer the pulp is in contact with the oral environment, the greater the risk of contamination. Primate experiments show that pulp capping may be carried out up to 24 hours after the pulp is exposed to the oral microflora. Usually, a thin film of fibrin and oral micro-organisms forms on the pulp surface which, within this time, can be washed off with simple lavage using sterile physiological saline. Subsequent pulp capping with calcium hydroxide promotes the formation of a calcific barrier provided that the whole is sealed with a restoration which prevents bacterial penetration to the pulp.

It is suggested, therefore, that pulp capping with calcium hydroxide is only carried out on the day of the injury (i.e. for practical purposes, within eight hours of the injury). This gives a generous margin in favour of a successful outcome.

(c) Degree of bacterial contamination

In the treatment of carious exposure of the pulp during cavity preparation, the pulp is either already contaminated by the oral microflora or becomes so almost immediately. Despite this, the pulp appears capable of overcoming a small degree of contamination. Pulp capping can be successful up to 24 hours after contamination although the longer the delay the slower the healing. It is essential to prevent re-contamination by ensuring that the restoration holding the pulp cap in place provides an effective seal.

(d) Associated injuries

The presence of concomitant luxation injury reduces the chance of successful treatment of the pulpal injury at the fracture surface. This is because the blood supply to the tooth is compromised by the damage to apical blood vessels particularly following intrusive or extrusive luxation. When treating teeth with multiple injuries, it is important to treat each injury on its merits and also warn the patient and parents of the reduced prognosis which can result from double injury.

2. Factors associated with treatment

(a) Presence of a blood clot

The presence of a blood clot between the medicament used to treat the exposed pulp and the vital pulp tissue itself reduces the incidence of healing and formation of a calcific barrier. It is thought that the clot and its degradation products interfere directly with healing, or that it acts as a barrier, preventing the therapeutic action of the medicament applied to the pulp. Blood clots, therefore, should either be removed or, when treatment involves operative procedures, prevented from forming. This may usually be achieved either by: (i) gentle irrigation with physiological saline immediately after operative procedures (e.g. pulpotomy); or (ii), when proposing to carry out a direct pulp capping procedure, removing the clot by gentle 'wiping' with a sterile cotton pledget moistened with sterile saline. Any further bleeding elicited is then controlled by gentle washing with sterile physiological saline until the bleeding stops by normal haemostatic mechanisms.

(b) Presence of inflammation

With regard to traumatized anterior teeth, the effects of pulpal inflammation on healing are poorly understood. In teeth with carious exposures the presence of inflammation is usually catastrophic. Even the placement of a calcium hydroxide medicament on to exposed pulp where the inflamed tissue has not been removed usually fails to prevent pulp death, with subsequent infection of the necrotic tissue and abscess formation. In so far as the aim of treatment of exposed pulps due to tooth crown fracture is the preservation of a vital, inflammation-free pulp, it is clear that removal of the inflamed part of the pulp is an important part of the management. In the traumatically exposed pulp it has been shown that, initially, inflammation affects only the outer 2 mm of the pulp. Removal of these superficial layers of pulp will reveal inflammation-free tissue which is likely to respond favourably to an appropriate medicament—usually calcium hydroxide.

(c) Operative technique and type of drill used

Techniques 2(minimal pulpotomy) and 3(cervical pulpotomy) (see pp. 48–51) involve increasing degrees of surgical intervention. The method used for amputation of coronal pulp tissue significantly influences healing. Three methods have been recommended: a spoon excavator; a steel bur at low speeds (conventional handpiece); and a diamond bur at very high speed (air-rotor). During pulp tissue removal the aim is to excise contaminated and inflamed tissue while causing minimal damage to the residual tissue.

The spoon excavator rarely cuts cleanly and tends to pull or stretch the residual pulp. It is probably the main cause of dystrophic calcification, especially in immature teeth. A slowly rotating steel bur inflicts significant injury to the residual pulp, reducing the chance of survival. This is probably because the cutting blades are inadequately controlled and fail to produce a 'clean' surgical cut. Nevertheless, an acceptable result may be obtained if the tissue amputation is carried out while steadying the cutting edges of the bur on a 'shelf' of dentine, cut at the same time as the pulp, with sterile physiological saline irrigating the pulp surface during cutting. A diamond bur in an air-rotor using a copious water spray enables a clean cut to be made with minimal damage to the remaining pulp.

It appears, therefore, that a careful surgical technique using diamond burs at high speed, well irrigated with sterile saline, which limits the impaction of dentine chips and creates a clean cut surface, is the technique of choice.

(d) Level of pulp amputation

The level of amputation *per se* is probably of little significance. Teeth treated by a partial or minimal pulpotomy and those by a full or cervical pulpotomy, all demonstrate excellent healing. The crucial factor seems to be the care taken in the cutting technique. Nevertheless, clinical reports do not give identical results, probably because the access necessary for a cervical pulpotomy is more difficult than the more superficial types of procedure. A significant advantage of the partial pulpotomy is maintenance of vital pulp in most of the crown of the tooth. In the cervical pulpotomy (see later), the crown of the tooth is effectively devitalized, becomes brittle and may, eventually, separate from the still vital root.

(e) Choice of pulp medicament

A wide range of materials has been used for pulp capping and related procedures and calcific barrier formation has been shown with many of them. The almost universal and successful use of calcium hydroxide means that, at present, there seems little justification for using other materials, although its mode of action is poorly understood. Some investigators state that the low solubility leads to a low concentration of hydroxyl ions, while others suggest that the dystrophic calcific barrier is laid down as a protection against the highly alkaline environment produced by calcium hydroxide. There seems little doubt that its high alkalinity also kills off any bacteria present, thereby improving the chances for uneventful healing.

Extensive experimental work has shown that following the application of a calcium hydroxide material to the pulp, well established changes take place. *Early reactions*: in the first 10 minutes three layers can be distinguished histologically. These are: I, a zone of compression: II, a zone of oedema and incipient liquefaction necrosis; III, a zone of intravascular coagulation necrosis. After six hours a further zone, IV, characterized by the appearance of polymorphonuclear lymphocytes is apparent. There is also a faint zone V detected as a faint fibrillar area delimiting zone IV. After 24 hours the borders between zones I, II, and III, are no longer apparent and zone IV is slightly more prominent. After seven days, new matrix forms in the area of zone IV, and zone V is no longer detectable. After three months the tissue formation in the place of zone IV resembles reparative dentine, with small dentine canals present. The superficial layers, formerly zones I, II, and III, have disintegrated into a thin layer of necrotic tissue. From about nine days the calcific barrier may be demonstrated radiographically.

The application of calcium hydroxide to vital pulp tissue results in a multilayered response leading to the differentiation of connective tissue and odontoblasts and the laying down of a calcific barrier.

Operative techniques for treating exposed pulp

The four techniques available for treating the exposed pulp are:

1. Direct pulp capping.
2. Minimal pulpotomy (partial pulpotomy/cornuectomy).
3. Cervical (radical) pulpotomy.
4. Pulpectomy.

1. Direct pulp capping

This is the procedure where an exposed dental pulp is covered with a dressing or cement in order to protect the pulp from additional injury and permit healing and repair (Fig. 4.12). With regard to fractured teeth it is the simplest of the four procedures. A calcium hydroxide preparation is used which may be a suspension or non-setting preparation such as Hypocal or a resin-based, rapid-setting material such as Dycal. Whichever is used, it is essential that it is held in place by a protective restoration (e.g. an etch-retained composite). If there is insufficient time at the emergency visit, or the patient is too distressed to co-operate adequately, the pulp capping material may be held in place with a layer of etch-retained fissure sealant or a glass ionomer cement. Such temporary restorations should be replaced by a definitive restoration after a few days—glass ionomer cements are particularly unreliable after 24 hours in these situations.

Results for direct pulp capping are somewhat equivocal: 72–88%, although there is some doubt about the case selection in some of the published studies. It is possible that some included teeth had also suffered luxation injury which would adversely affect healing because of interference with the blood supply to the pulp. Nevertheless, direct pulp capping in teeth which have suffered no other injury provides a simple and frequently effective treatment with a success rate comparable to that for the minimal (partial) pulpotomy.

The main disadvantages of direct pulp capping are the difficulty of ensuring that no blood clot is left on the surface of the exposed pulp, which is known to interfere with healing by promoting inflammation, and the danger of sealing in bacteria between the medicament and the pulp, which may cause inflammation and failure of healing.

Technique of direct pulp capping

Clinical conditions required:

(a) the pulp should be free from inflammation due to previous injury or caries;

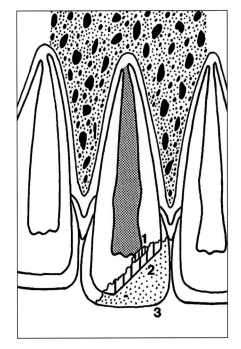

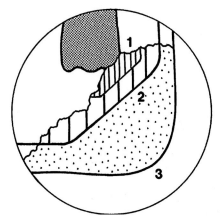

Fig. 4.12 Schematic representation of direct pulp capping to treat a coronal fracture involving enamel, dentine, and pulp: (1) calcium hydroxide on exposed pulp tissue; (2) calcium hydroxide on surrounding dentine; (3) etch-retained composite restoration.

(b) there should be no associated damage to apical blood vessels from a luxation injury;

(c) the same day as the injury;

(d) an immature or a mature tooth.

Clinical technique:

(a) isolate tooth;

(b) gently remove any blood clot with a sterile cotton pellet moistened with sterile saline;

(c) gently dry around the exposure site with sterile cotton pellets;

(d) apply a calcium hydroxide medicament (e.g. Hypocal or Dycal) (Fig. 4.12, 1);

(e) apply a setting calcium hydroxide cement (e.g. Dycal) to the exposed dentine (Fig. 4.12, 2);

(f) apply the protective restoration (Fig. 4.12, 3);

(g) if a temporary protective restoration has been used this should be replaced by a definitive restoration after a few days;

(h) review the patient after three months.

2. Minimal pulpotomy (partial pulpotomy/cornuectomy)

This the procedure where part of the superficial coronal pulp is removed in order to eliminate inflamed and contaminated tissue that has been exposed to the oral cavity. The pulp wound is then dressed with a calcium hydroxide preparation in order to protect the pulp from further injury and permit healing and repair (Fig. 4.13). The calcium hydroxide preparation again may be a suspension or non-setting preparation such as Hypocal, or a resin-based, rapid-setting material such as Dycal. Whichever is used, it is essential that it is held in place by a protective restoration (e.g. an etch-retained composite). On the basis of the experimental studies previously described, the depth of pulp which should be removed is usually 2–3 mm. The amount of pulp removed laterally is governed by the pulp anatomy at the exposure site but usually results in a larger pulp wound.

This technique gives excellent results, 96% success when carried out according to the technique described by Cvek (1978), and may be used for teeth which have been fractured up to 72 hours previously. Many operators use it in preference to direct pulp capping as there is a more certain outcome because the technique ensures that blood clot and bacteria are not allowed to come between the calcium hydroxide medicament and the pulp tissue.

Technique for minimal pulpotomy

Clinical conditions required:

(a) the pulp should be free from inflammation due to previous injury or caries;

(b) there should be no associated damage to apical blood vessels from a luxation injury;

(c) the time since the accident may be up to 72 hours;

(d) an immature or a mature tooth.

Figure 4.14 is a radiograph of a 10-year-old girl who had fractured the crowns of 11 and 21 with pulp exposure. The teeth were immature and were treated by minimal pulpotomy.

Clinical technique:

(a) anaesthetize the tooth (inhalation sedation may be helpful for very anxious patients);

(b) isolate the tooth;

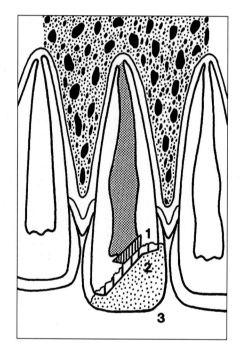

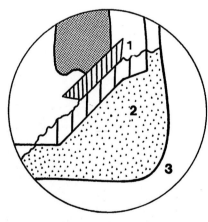

Fig. 4.13 Schematic representation of minimal pulpotomy to treat a coronal fracture involving enamel, dentine, and pulp: (1) calcium hydroxide applied to the pulp wound after preparation; (2) calcium hydroxide cement on surrounding dentine; (3) etch-retained composite restoration.

(c) prepare a cavity at the exposure site, 2–3 mm deep and 2–4 mm wide using an air-rotor with a diamond bur, ensuring copious irrigation;

(d) gently irrigate the prepared cavity with physiological saline until the bleeding stops—usually within 7–8 minutes. If the bleeding does not stop after 10 minutes, more extensive inflammation has developed and a cervical pulpotomy (see below) will probably be necessary;

(e) blot the cavity dry with sterile paper points, taking care not to touch the pulp and cause further bleeding (Fig. 4.15);

(f) place calcium hydroxide in the base of the cavity (Fig. 4.16), with a further layer to fill the cavity and extend it to cover the dentine surrounding the amputation site (Fig. 4.17);

(g) restore the tooth with an etch-retained composite, which also protects the calcium hydroxide;

(h) review the patient after three months, six months, and at their routine dental check-ups thereafter.

The radiograph in Fig. 4.18 shows the successful outcome two years after the original injury with the completion of root development of 11 and healthy periapical tissues.

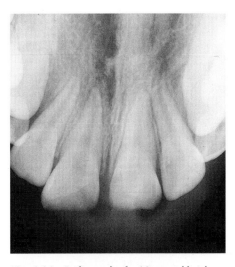

Fig. 4.14 Radiograph of a 10-year-old girl. Upper central incisors (immature) were fractured involving enamel, dentine, and pulp.

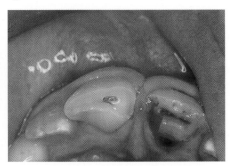

Fig. 4.15 Minimal pulpotomy has been carried out on 11, bleeding has stopped and calcium hydroxide is to be applied.

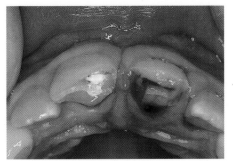

Fig. 4.16 Calcium hydroxide applied to the pulp at the amputation site of 11.

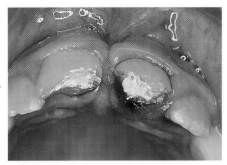

Fig. 4.17 Calcium hydroxide applied to remaining dentine surrounding the amputation site of 11.

3. Cervical (radical) pulpotomy

This is the procedure where the complete coronal pulp is removed to the constriction in the root canal, which is the anatomical junction of the crown and root of the tooth. Again, the pulp surface is dressed with a calcium hydroxide preparation to protect the pulp from further injury and permit healing and repair (Fig. 4.19). The technique, whose objective is also to maintain the vitality of the pulp in an immature tooth so that root development continues to maturity, has been part of clinical practice for many decades. It was customary, once root development was complete, to root fill the tooth and prepare and fit a post–crown. More recently, root filling has been considered to be unnecessary until or unless the root canal is needed to support a restoration. As the success rate for cervical pulpotomy is a relatively modest 72% compared to a 96% success rate for minimal pulpotomy, the latter technique is preferred. The minimal pulpotomy also has the added advantage that almost all the coronal pulp remains vital and, therefore, avoids brittleness and later coronal fracture.

Nevertheless, cervical pulpotomy has a small but important part to play. If other treatment has been unsuccessful or when there has been significant delay in the provision of treatment resulting in prolonged exposure to the oral cavity and impaction of debris, inflammation will have spread further into the pulp. In these circumstances, a more extensive removal of pulp tissue will be required if

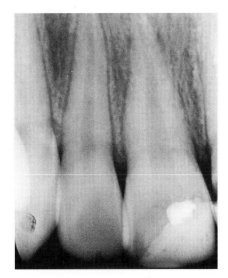

Fig. 4.18 Radiograph of 11 (same patient as in Figs 4.14–4.17) two years after the minimal pulpotomy showing a successful outcome with completion of root growth and healthy periapical tissues.

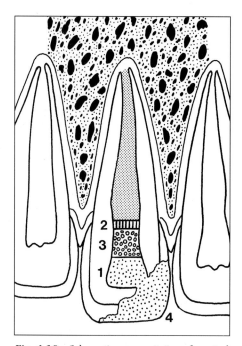

Fig. 4.19 Schematic representation of cervical pulpotomy to treat a coronal fracture involving enamel, dentine, and pulp: (2) calcium hydroxide; (3) polycarboxylate cement; (1 and 4) etch-retained composite.

healthy tissue is to be reached on to which the calcium hydroxide medicament may be placed. In the case shown in Fig. 4.20, both upper central incisors were fractured three days previously, the fractures involving enamel, dentine, and pulp (Fig. 4.21).

Technique of cervical (radical) pulpotomy

Clinical conditions required:

(a) immature tooth (Fig. 4.22);

(b) pulp inflammation has penetrated more deeply than 2 mm;

(c) usually more than 72 hours since the injury;

(d) no luxation injury.

Clinical technique:

(a) anaesthetize the tooth (inhalation sedation may be helpful for very anxious patients);

(b) isolate the tooth;

(c) gain access to the pulp chamber using a high-speed handpiece and diamond bur with copious irrigation and amputate the pulp at the level of the cervical constriction;

(d) gently irrigate the pulp surface with physiological saline until the bleeding stops—7–8 minutes. If the bleeding is persistent it may be necessary to carry out a complete pulp extirpation and subsequently treat the tooth in the same way as a non-vital immature tooth (see Chapter 7);

(f) blot the pulp chamber dry, taking care not to touch the pulp and cause further bleeding (Fig. 4.23);

(g) place a calcium hydroxide paste on the radicular pulp (use calcium hydroxide powder with sterile water or a proprietary preparation (e.g. Hypocal) (Fig. 4.24);

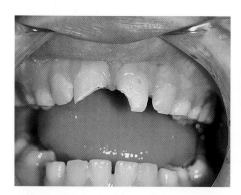

Fig. 4.20 Permanent upper central incisors (11, 21) fractured three days previously in an 8-year-old child.

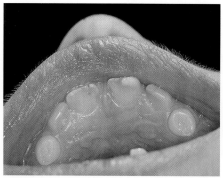

Fig. 4.21 Same patient as in Fig. 4.20, showing exposed pulp of 11. The pulp of 21 was also exposed but does not show clearly in this view.

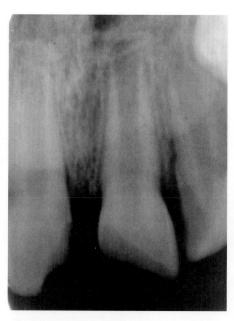

Fig. 4.22 Same patient: radiograph of 11, 21 showing immature root form.

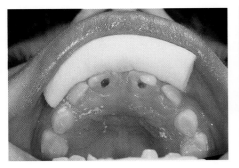

Fig. 4.23 Same patient: coronal pulp has been removed and bleeding has ceased.

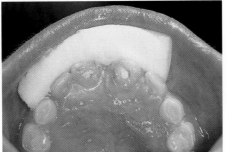

Fig. 4.24 Calcium hydroxide placed on amputated pulp.

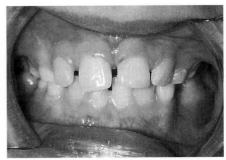

Fig. 4.25 Fractured 11, 21 restored with etch-retained composite after pulpotomies have been completed.

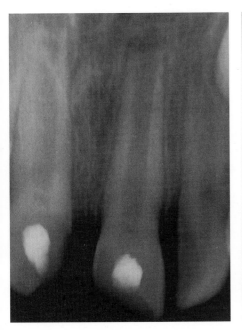

Fig. 4.26 Radiograph of 11, 21, six weeks after the pulpotomies showing early calcific barrier formation

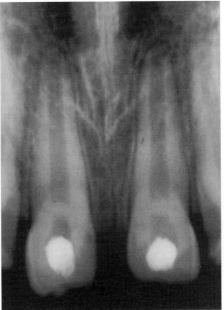

Fig. 4.27 Radiograph of 11, 21, one year after the pulpotomies showing well-formed calcific barriers and continued root development.

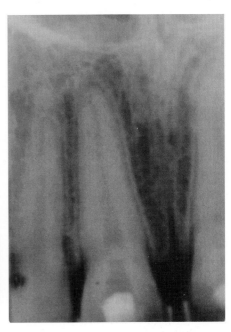

Fig. 4.28 Radiograph of 11, 21, ten years after the pulpotomies showing mature root anatomy.

(h) seal the access cavity with zinc phosphate or polycarboxylate cement and restore with etch-retained composite (Fig. 4.25);

(i) review the patient—usually after three months, six months, and annually thereafter.

The radiographs in Figs 4.26, 4.27, and 4.28 are of the patient illustrated in Figs 4.20–4.25, 6 weeks, one year, and 10 years post-pulpotomy.

4. Pulpectomy

This is the complete removal of the dental pulp. It is usually indicated when the tooth is mature (i.e. in children older than 13–14 years of age); when the pulpal exposure is more than 8 hours old; and/or when there is an associated luxation injury with probable damage to the apical blood vessels. A common assumption is that by 10–11 years of age, upper permanent incisors have a mature root with

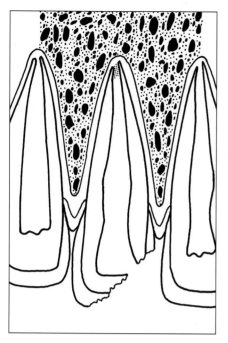

Fig. 4.29 Schematic representation of essentially mature tooth prior to root canal therapy.

a constricted apical foramen. This is rarely true. Confusion is caused by the fact that on intra-oral radiographs, which show only the mesio-distal dimension, the root frequently appears mature with a fairly narrow canal and apical constriction. However, at this age the root canal is oval, with an incomplete apical foramen, but as the 'ovality' is bucco-palatal it cannot be seen on the usual intra-oral radiograph. Conventional root filling of the tooth at this stage is likely to be unsuccessful because of the difficulty in obtaining a satisfactory apical seal. (The situation of the immature non-vital tooth is discussed fully in Chapter 7.)

Clinical technique for pulpectomy
Clinical conditions required:

(a) mature tooth (Fig. 4.29);
(b) exposure present for longer than 8 hours;
(c) possible damage to apical blood vessels due to associated luxation injury.

Clinical technique:

(a) anaesthetize the tooth (inhalation sedation] may be helpful for very anxious patients);
(b) isolate tooth;
(c) gain access to the pulp chamber using a long, tapered diamond bur in an air-rotor;
(d) extirpate the pulp with a barbed broach. A pre-operative long cone periapical radiograph (Fig. 4.30) will provide a good, initial, guide to root length;
(e) place a fine reamer, file, or gutta percha point (Fig. 4.31) in the canal to the estimated length and take a further radiograph to establish an accurate working length;
(f) file the canal to the appropriate length until clean dentine is obtained. Irrigate the canal with sodium hypochlorite solution followed by sterile saline and dry with paper points.
(g) dress the canal with antibiotic paste or non-setting calcium hydroxide paste for one week;
(h) when orthodontic treatment is proposed, a provisional root filling of non-setting calcium is maintained until tooth movements have been completed. The calcium hydroxide should be replenished every 6 to 8 months;
(i) at the appropriate time complete the root filling with laterally condensed multiple gutta percha points and root canal sealer (Fig. 4.32).

TREATMENT OF MULTIPLE INJURIES

A patient may present with several injuries involving the same tooth. The priority is to ensure that an accurate diagnosis has been made so that the most important injury is treated first (e.g. extrusive luxation is treated before an exposed pulp). The presence of more than one injury usually reduces the prognosis and it is prudent to advise the patient and/or parents of this.

CROWN–ROOT FRACTURES

A further complication to coronal fracture involving enamel and dentine, and enamel, dentine and pulp is when part of the fracture line passes beneath the gingival margin. This may be a vertical fracture or more oblique. The extent of

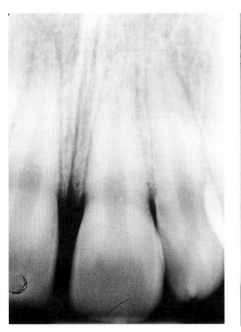

Fig. 4.30 Non-vital 21 prior to root canal therapy.

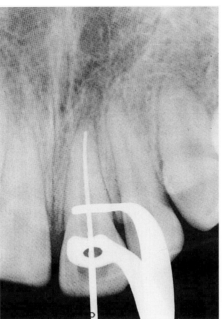

Fig. 4.31 Non-vital 21 with diagnostic instrument in root canal during root canal therapy.

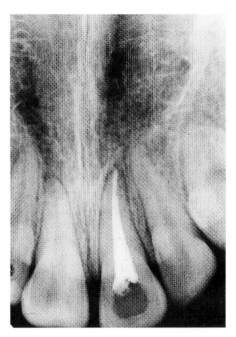

Fig. 4.32 Non-vital 21 with completed root filling.

the fracture beneath the gingival margin is often difficult to determine at first. However, as treatment will usually involve removing the loose fragment which is often held in close apposition to the rest of the tooth by the periodontal ligament fibres, some assessment of the apical extent of the fracture can be made by inspecting the removed fragment and/or the tooth itself.

In general, although the treatment can be difficult in terms of long-term restoration, initial care will follow the same principles described in the preceding sections on coronal fracture. It is often sufficient to restore the supragingival aspect in the usual way but leave the subgingival aspect untreated until most of the child's growing has been achieved. At that time a number of cases will have resolved in that the fracture will now be completely supragingival, due to continued eruption. Where this has not happened (usually the more extensive fractures) it can then be decided if the tooth can be extruded orthodontically to achieve the same result, or whether a surgical approach will be required to gain access to the most apical part of the fracture line prior to placement of a restoration.

FURTHER READING

Andreasen, J. O. and Andreasen, F. M. (1990). *Essentials of traumatic injuries to the teeth.* Munksgaard, Copenhagen.

Andreasen, J. O. and Andreasen, F. M. (1994).*Textbook and color atlas of traumatic injuries to the teeth,* (3rd edn). Munksgaard, Copenhagen.

Cvek, M. (1978). A clinical report on partial pulpotomy and capping with calcium hydroxide in permanent incisors with complicated crown fracture. *Journal of Endodontology,* **4**, 232–7.

Friend, L. A. (1967). Root canal morphology in incisor teeth in the 6–15 year old child. *International Endodontology Journal,* **10**, 35–42.

Hallet, G. E. and Porteous, J. R. (1963). Fractured incisors treated by vital pulpotomy. A report on 100 consecutive cases. *British Dental Journal,* **115**, 279–87.

5 Root fracture

5 Root fracture

ROOT fracture is rare, accounting for an estimated 1% of all tooth injuries, with a range of 0.5–7% (See Table 1.1). Although the fracture involves cementum, dentine, and pulp, the majority of teeth damaged in this way retain a vital pulp. In one large study, healing was observed in 74% of cases, failure of healing with loss of pulp vitality in 26%. As a large number of the patients in the study were adults with mature teeth, it is reasonable to expect the relatively immature teeth of the younger age group to have a better outcome in this respect. It appears that the pulp in the apical portion of a root fractured tooth almost invariably remains vital.

CLINICAL PRESENTATION AND DIAGNOSIS

Root fractures, luxation injuries, and fractures of the alveolar process frequently have a similar clinical presentation—mobility and/or displacement. The correct diagnosis of a root fracture relies on the use of appropriate radiographs. The labio-palatal angulation of fracture lines varies greatly, from high (apical) labially and low (gingival) palatally to low labially and high palatally. Truly horizontal fractures are found most frequently near the cervical (gingival) region of the tooth (Fig. 5.1). A blow which causes root fracture will usually also result in some degree of luxation of the coronal fragment. The same terminology is used as for luxation injuries without associated root fracture (Fig. 5.2), although it is extremely rare to find an intrusive luxation superimposed on a root fracture. Concussion accounts for 3% of cases; subluxation 21%; extrusion 37%; lateral luxation 39%.

RADIOGRAPHS

The great variation in angulation of root fractures means that two radiographs, taken at different angles to the long axis of the tooth, are usually required to confirm or refute the provisional clinical diagnosis. In Fig. 5.3, the injured tooth (11) appeared satisfactory. However, one month later, a further radiograph revealed a root fracture (Fig. 5.4) when, perhaps, the angulation of the X-ray beam was different and the fragments had separated further. Another complicating factor is that any change in the orientation of the X-ray beam relative to the long axis of the tooth alters the radiographic appearance of the fracture. This is well illustrated in Figs 5.5 and 5.6: in the first film the fracture appears as a single, thin line, while in the second there appear to be two fracture lines. This is explained by the fact that in the first film, the X-ray beam is at the same angle to the long axis of the tooth as the fracture itself, while in the second the beam is at a quite a different angle to the fracture and the buccal and palatal aspects of the fracture are projected separately.

When no other injuries are suspected, an anterior occlusal view and an intra-oral periapical view are taken and may be expected to reveal 98% of root frac-

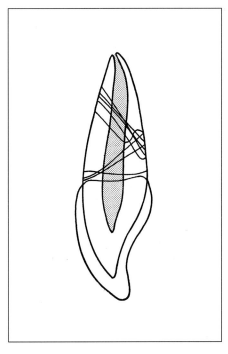

Fig. 5.1 Direction and angulation of fracture lines in root fracture in permanent upper central incisor teeth. (After Andreasen 1981.)

CONCUSSION **SUBLUXATION** **EXTRUSION** **LATERAL LUXATION**

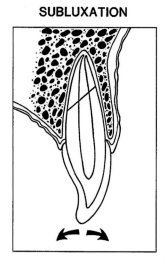
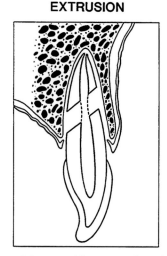
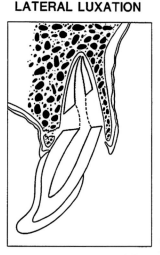

Fig. 5.2 Luxation injuries of the coronal fragments of root fractures in permanent incisors. (After Andreasen and Andreasen 1988.)

tures. The intra-oral periapical view is ideally taken using the long cone technique. However, when the long cone technique cannot be used, perhaps because pain from soft tissue injury prevents the patient tolerating the film holder or the patient has difficulty opening their mouth, the bisecting angle technique will suffice.

Root fractures have commonly been designated as being in the apical, middle or coronal third of the root. However, the dividing lines are essentially arbitrary and often have little bearing on the outcome. In general, it may be said that the closer the fracture is to the apex, the better the prognosis.

In young people, root fracture is particularly uncommon perhaps because the immature root form and more elastic bone makes these teeth more susceptible to luxation injury than fracture.

VITALITY TESTING

Vitality testing of root fractured teeth soon after injury will provide an indication of the likelihood of long-term maintenance of pulp vitality or the subsequent development of pulp necrosis. In one large study of adults, adolescents and children, a positive result at initial presentation was usually associated with continuing pulp vitality, while a negative result indicated a one-in-three chance of subsequent pulp necrosis and associated failure of healing.

Pulp canal obliteration, affecting the coronal fragment, is a common sequel to root fracture—73% in one large study. A reduced response to conventional vitality testing will be, therefore, an expected finding in teeth where pulp canal obliteration has affected the coronal fragment.

TREATMENT

The overall aim of treatment is to preserve pulp vitality whenever possible and to restore the integrity of the relationship of the root fragments and that of the root and the alveolar bone.

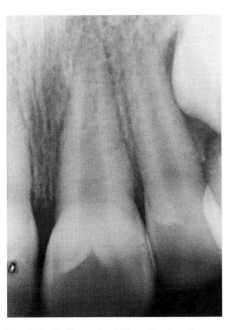

Fig. 5.3 Radiograph of 21 on the day of injury. No hard tissue injury was noted.

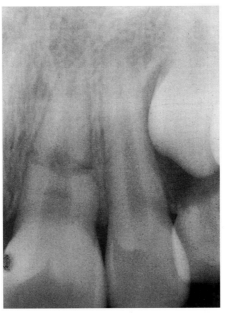

Fig. 5.4 Radiograph of 21 (same patient as in Fig. 5.3) one month later, showing a root fracture, perhaps because of a slightly different angulation of the X-ray beam and separation of the fragments.

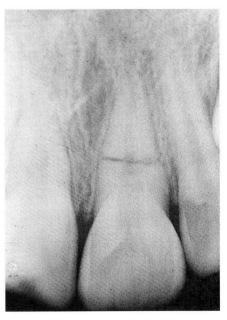

Fig. 5.5 Slightly foreshortened periapical radiograph of 21 showing the root fracture as a single line.

Objectives of treatment

(1) to encourage hard tissue union between the root fragments;

(2) to maintain pulp vitality;

(3) to allow completion of root growth and maturation (immature teeth).

These objectives may be achieved by:

(a) reduction of the fracture;

(b) splinting for 12 weeks;

(c) regular follow-up—routine vitality testing and occasional radiographs.

Reduction of the fracture

The fracture is reduced by firm digital pressure on the incisal edge of the crown of the tooth. Local analgesia may, or may not, be necessary usually depending on how mobile the coronal fragment is and how severely displaced.

If difficulty is experienced when repositioning the coronal fragment, this may be because the bone of the socket wall has been displaced or the patient has presented late, when consolidation and tissue repair at the fracture site is already advanced. In the former, it may be possible to reposition the displaced bone using a small flat instrument placed in the socket and then reducing the fracture as previously described. In the latter situation, it may not be possible to reduce the fracture completely.

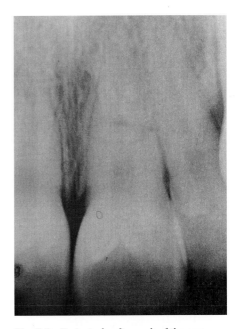

Fig. 5.6 Periapical radiograph of the same tooth as Fig. 5.5, taken at a different angle, apparently showing a double fracture of the root.

Splinting

Splinting allows the coronal fragment to be maintained in a 'normal' anatomical relationship to the apical fragment. Successful maintenance of this relationship will encourage healing and union of the apical and coronal fragments. When complete reduction is not possible it may be necessary to adjust the occlusion to relieve premature contact between the damaged tooth and the opposing teeth.

The appropriate splinting period for root fractures is 12 weeks. During this time, regular clinical assessment, vitality tests, and, possibly, radiological examination will be needed so that should endodontic therapy become necessary, it may be started as soon as possible. After 12 weeks the splint is removed and the tooth assessed for colour, mobility, and vitality.

PRELIMINARY TISSUE CHANGES

Root fracture causes a variable degree of damage to the dental pulp and the periodontal structures close to the fracture line, which results in bleeding in the pulp and periodontium. A coagulum forms in and around the fracture line, its size depending on the extent of separation of the fragments. After a few days, proliferating odontoblasts may be detected entering the fracture line and over the next few weeks a dentine callus develops. Within a month, cementum is deposited on the outer surface of the root fragments and the major part of the fracture line is filled with connective tissue. Although there are similarities with the repair process seen in bone fractures, repair of tooth root fracture takes place much more slowly. This is because of the low vascularity of the area compared to bone and because dentine, unlike bone, does not undergo constant remodelling. Following these preliminary changes, healing of two main types may take place, or there may be failure of healing.

The type of healing subsequently found probably depends on the extent of any displacement of the fragments and also on the success, or otherwise, of repositioning and splinting. The maturity of the tooth also has a significant influence on the potential for healing, immature teeth having much better healing properties than mature teeth.

HEALING

Two main types of healing may be identified:

Type I   Healing with hard tissue.

Type II   Healing with ingrowth of connective tissue or with ingrowth of bone and connective tissue.

The two aspects of healing in Type II are sometimes considered as two distinct conditions but they are really variants of the same healing process and will, therefore, be considered as a single entity here.

Type I healing: healing with hard tissue

Approximately one-third of all root fractured teeth exhibit healing with hard tissue union, the coronal and apical fragments being united by external deposition of cementum, internal deposition of dentine and by both cementum and dentine growing into the fracture line to a greater or lesser extent (Fig. 5.7). Histologically, the hard tissue in the fracture line is not solid but interspersed with connective tissue which reduces its radiopacity, so that the fracture line often remains visible on radiographs.

Root fractures in teeth with immature roots are uncommon. This is probably because of the relative elasticity of the alveolar bone in young patients which

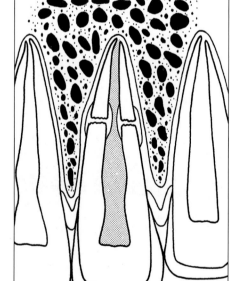

Fig. 5.7 Schematic representation of healing of a root fracture: external deposition of cementum, internal deposition of dentine, and growth of both tissues into the fracture line.

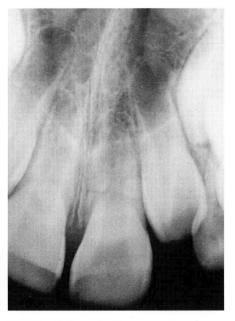

Fig. 5.8 Radiograph of immature 21 with root fracture

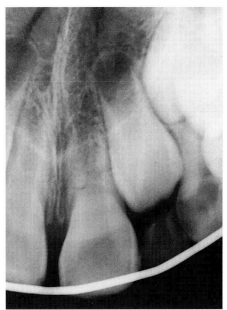

Fig. 5.9 Radiograph of immature 21 (same patient as in Fig. 5.8) after reduction of root fracture and provision of an etch-retained splint.

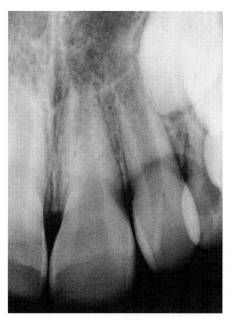

Fig. 5.10 Radiograph of 21 (same patient as in Figs 5.8, 5.9) two years after original injury. Root fracture has healed and root development has continued.

tends to make luxation injury more likely than root fracture. When fracture does take place the thin, immature, root canal wall undergoes what is comparable to a greenstick fracture seen in the bones of children (Fig. 5.8). The fragments are usually only slightly displaced and, therefore, easy to reduce (Fig. 5.9). Immobilization is most readily achieved with an etch-retained composite and stainless steel wire splint. However, a removable splint, rather like a removable orthodontic appliance, may be the only option if there are no suitable adjacent teeth to anchor the etch-retained splint to—quite common in the early mixed dentition. Two years later there has been continued root development, so that the healed fracture has become incorporated in the new root tissue. The only remaining evidence is the narrowing of the pulp canal in the region of the original fracture site (Fig. 5.10). Four years after the original injury, the tooth has grown almost normally and, apart from the dentine callus in the root canal, appears unaffected. Continued, essentially normal root development is a feature of root fracture in immature teeth (Fig. 5.11).

External surface root resorption, which rounds off the sharp edges of the fracture in more mature teeth, has been described in 28% of root fractures healing by hard tissue union, the resorption being observed before the reparative hard tissue is laid down. In a further 34%, a similar pattern of resorption of the internal fracture surfaces was also described and internal tunnelling resorption in 6% of cases. Unlike the resorption seen as a complication of intrusive, extrusive and, total luxation (avulsion), that seen following root fracture is usually quite minimal, the lost tissue quickly becoming replaced by the hard tissues of the healing process. Evidence of this type of resorption is not a signal for embarking on endodontic therapy!

Calcification of the pulp, seen on serial radiographs as a progressive narrowing of the root canal, is a common response in root fractured teeth (73% of teeth in one study) and frequently leads to obliteration of the pulp canal. It may involve the canal of the apical fragment alone, the coronal fragment alone or both apical and coronal fragments. In teeth with Type I healing, pulp canal obliteration is almost as frequently seen in the apical fragment alone (44%) as in the coronal

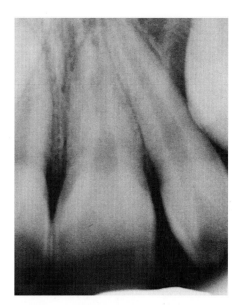

Fig. 5.11 Radiograph of 21 (same patient) four years after original injury showing continued root maturation after healing.

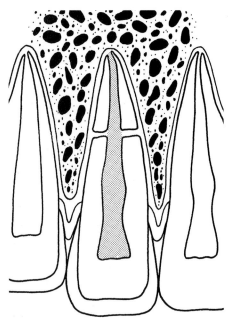

Fig. 5.12 Schematic representation of Type II healing with interposition of connective tissue between the fragments.

and apical fragments combined (48%) but is infrequent in the coronal fragment alone (approximately 7%).

Hard tissue union is the most desirable outcome and is likely to be more common in less mature teeth where there is a good blood supply and good healing potential. Once the hard tissue union has consolidated, the tooth may again be treated as a single entity, although care should be exercised if orthodontic treatment is undertaken, especially if strong torquing forces are employed.

Type II healing: healing with ingrowth of connective tissue, or connective tissue and bone

Forty per cent of root fractured teeth exhibit healing with the interposition of connective tissue, or connective tissue and bone, between the fragments (Fig. 5.12). This is a good outcome and usually causes no further problems, although there will be a moderate degree of residual mobility in many cases.

An example of Type II healing, with ingrowth of connective tissue between the fragments, is shown in Fig. 5.13 where, in these early stages of healing, some resorption of the jagged edges of the fractured dentine is also apparent. Secondary dentine formation has formed a new 'apical' foramen at the fracture line: the so-called 'fracture foramen'. Radiographically the rounding of the sharp dentine edges can be seen with a thin radiolucent line separating the two edges (Figs 5.13, 5.14). This rounding of the sharp edges is the result of the same type of resorption as previously described for teeth healing with hard tissue union.

In the case illustrated in Figs 5.15 and 5.16, there is ingrowth of bone, as well as connective tissue, between the apical and coronal fragments. This type of healing is associated with the normal dento-alveolar growth and development that takes place in children. The apical fragment apparently remains in its original position while the coronal fragment continues to erupt, together with the adjacent teeth. Root resorption is also evident in this case.

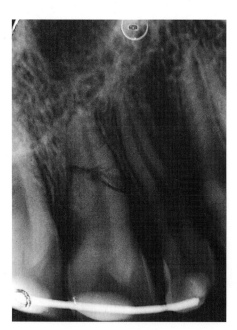

Fig. 5.13 Root fracture of 21, one year after injury, showing Type II healing. Secondary dentine has caused a slight constriction of the root canal just coronal to the fracture, forming the 'fracture foramen'.

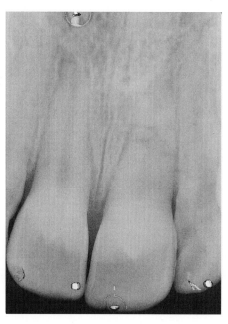

Fig. 5.14 Same patient as in Fig. 5.13, two years later. In addition to the Type II healing previously noted there has been progressive pulp canal obliteration affecting the coronal and apical fragments.

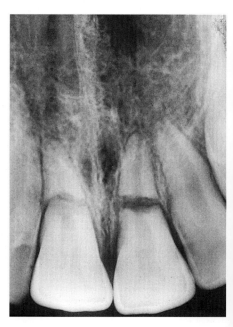

Fig. 5.15 Radiograph of 11, 21 which have both suffered root fracture.

In fact, all three types of root resorption seen in root fractures showing Type I healing are also seen in cases of Type II healing, but with a greater prevalence: 61% show external surface root resorption, 58% show internal surface resorption, and 37% internal tunnelling resorption. Again, unlike the resorption seen as a complication of luxation injuries including avulsion, that seen in Type II healing following root fracture is usually quite minimal, the lost tissue quickly becoming replaced by the hard tissues of the healing process.

A similar pattern of pulp canal obliteration to that described for cases with Type I healing is also seen in Type II healing although, as with the resorption, there are differences, pulp canal calcification being much more commonly seen in apical and coronal fragments combined (73%) as compared to apical (17%) or coronal (10%) alone. Total or partial obliteration of both coronal and apical fragment root canals may be seen in the case illustrated in Fig. 5.16. (It is also apparent in the case illustrated in Fig 5.14.)

In all cases of Type II healing, while the teeth may usually be considered to be 'normal' in most respects, their shortened roots may make them more prone to avulsion in subsequent traumatic episodes. Also, orthodontic movement of root fractured teeth which show healing with ingrowth of connective tissue alone may lead to disengagement of the fragments or unpredictable resorption. When there has been healing with ingrowth of both connective tissue and bone, orthodontic movement will frequently result in further separation of the fragments although intrusive movement will tend to approximate the fragments and may also cause unpredictable resorption.

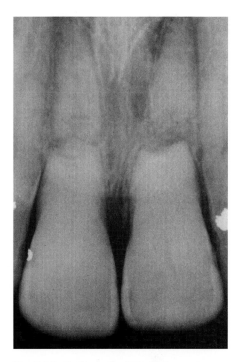

Fig. 5.16 Radiograph of 11, 21 (same case as in Fig. 5.15) 18 months after original injury, showing Type II healing with ingrowth of bone and connective tissue. The coronal fragment has continued to erupt while the apical fragment has apparently stayed in its original position. Root canal obliteration affects both teeth in both apical and coronal fragments.

FAILURE OF HEALING

When all age groups are considered, failure of healing affects approximately one quarter of all root fractured teeth and is associated with necrosis of the pulp in the coronal fragment, although the apical fragment almost invariably retains its vitality. However, in the immature roots of younger patients pulp necrosis is a much less common complication, presumably because of the very good blood supply and potential for repair and further development.

The necrotic pulp of the coronal fragment eventually becomes infected and infection spreads from the root canal to affect the adjacent alveolar bone (Fig. 5.17). Clinically, there will often be inflammation of the mucosa overlying the root; sometimes the presence of a sinus, usually at the level of the fracture rather than over the apex; increased mobility of the tooth and tenderness—the typical signs of an infected, necrotic pulp. The radiographic appearance in failure of healing is characterized by radiolucency in the bone adjacent to the fracture line often associated with displacement of the apical fragment by the expanding area of infection (Fig. 5.18). Interestingly, obliteration of the pulp canal in the apical fragment is a feature of most cases when there is failure of healing. However, as this form of calcification can only take place where there is healthy, vital pulp tissue, pulp canal obliteration is not seen in the coronal fragment in cases of failed healing.

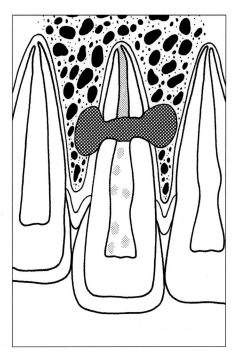

Fig. 5.17 Schematic representation of failure of healing showing the spread of infection from the root canal of the coronal fragment into the bone adjacent to the fracture line.

TREATMENT

The management of a root fractured tooth which has failed to heal is directed at controlling the infection associated with the necrotic pulp tissue in the coronal fragment.

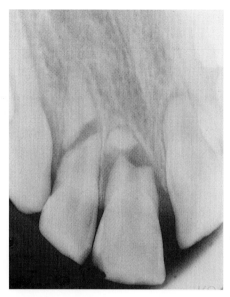

Fig. 5.18 Failure of healing: radiograph of 12, 11 showing radiolucency at the fracture line of each tooth and some displacement of the apical fragments following necrosis and infection affecting the pulps of the coronal fragments.

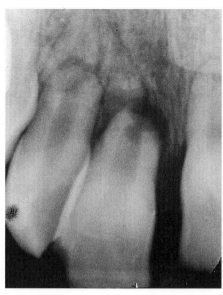

Fig. 5.19 Radiograph of the case in Fig. 5.18 revealing further deterioration in the condition of 12 and 11. 11 was unsaveable and, therefore, extracted. Endodontic therapy was carried out on 12 (see Fig. 5.20).

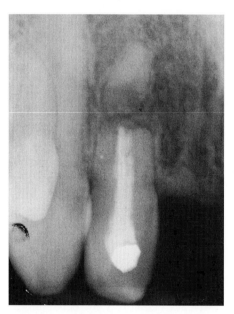

Fig. 5.20 Radiograph of 12 showing root filling to the fracture line (same patient as in Fig. 5.18 and 5.19).

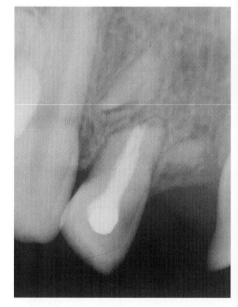

Fig. 5.21 Radiograph of 12 after one year showing resolution of the infection and subsequent healing with ingrowth of connective tissue and bone (same patient as in Figs 5.18–5.20).

A case of failure of healing is illustrated in Figs 5.18 and 5.19. Clinically, the coronal fragments of these teeth were mobile, slightly extruded from their sockets, tender to percussion, and failed to respond to routine vitality testing. The upper right central incisor was unsaveable and was, therefore, extracted. Conventional root canal therapy to the fracture foramen of the upper right lateral incisor (Fig. 5.20) resulted in resolution of the infection and subsequent healing by ingrowth of connective tissue and bone between the root fragments (Fig. 5.21).

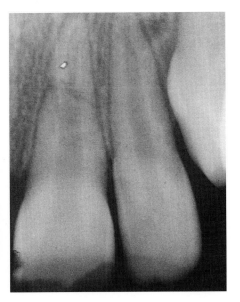

Fig. 5.22 Radiograph of 21 showing oblique angle of root fracture.

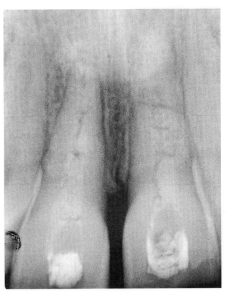

Fig. 5.23 Radiograph of 21 showing root canal obturated with calcium hydroxide to the fracture foramen only. The 11 was non-vital, immature, but with no root fracture. The whole canal was obturated with calcium hydroxide (same patient as in Fig. 5.22).

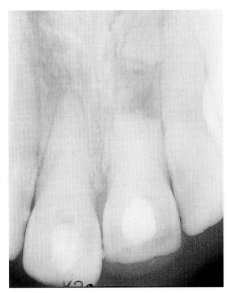

Fig. 5.24 Radiograph of 21 (same patient as in Figs 5.22, 5.23) two years later. The infection has resolved with hard tissue barrier formation at the fracture foramen. The tooth was then root filled to this barrier at the fracture line (Fig. 5.25).

However, one problem which may be encountered is the abnormal shape of the fracture foramen when the fracture line is oblique (see Fig. 5.1). In such a case (Fig. 5.22), it is extremely difficult to instrument the canal to obtain the 'apical stop' just within the fracture foramen required for satisfactorily filling the root canal. This problem may be overcome by removing the necrotic debris from the root canal and, following thorough mechanical cleansing, irrigation, and drying, obturating the canal to the fracture foramen with calcium hydroxide (Fig. 5.23). The calcium hydroxide should be changed at six–eight month intervals. In due course, as the infection resolves and there is healing, a hard tissue barrier forms at the fracture foramen (Fig. 5.24), facilitating the placement of a permanent root filling (Fig. 5.25).

ORTHODONTIC TREATMENT FOR HEALED ROOT FRACTURED TEETH

Teeth that have undergone Type I healing may be regarded as essentially normal. However, it is prudent to delay active orthodontic movement of such teeth until approximately 12 months have elapsed since the injury. This allows for the three-month splinting period, plus six months to allow resolution of any resorptive processes, plus a further three months as a 'safety margin'.

Figure 5.26 shows a root fracture of 11 in a 9-year-old boy. Partial reduction was achieved and the tooth splinted using an orthodontic bracket and wire (Fig. 5.27). After 12 weeks, the splint was removed and the tooth rested for a period of a year. The tooth was then incorporated in an appliance to reduce the overjet (Fig. 5.28), and five years later is in a good position, of good colour, with pulp canal obliteration of both coronal and apical fragments (Fig. 5.29).

As has been mentioned previously, in Type II healing, orthodontic movement may cause separation of the fragments when there has been healing with ingrowth of connective tissue or, in intrusive movement, unpredictable resorption. When there has been healing with ingrowth of both bone and connective

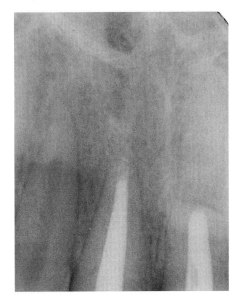

Fig. 5.25 Radiograph of 21 showing completed root filling to the fracture foramen barrier (same patient as in Figs 5.22–5.24). 11 has also had its permanent root filling placed.

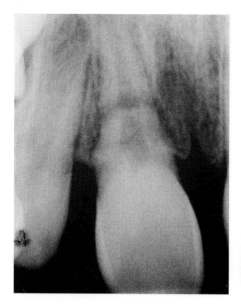

Fig. 5.26 Radiograph of 11 showing root fracture in a 9-year-old boy.

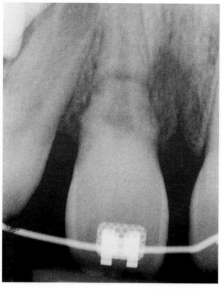

Fig. 5.27 Radiograph of 11 (same patient as in Fig. 5.26) three months later. The tooth had been splinted with an orthodontic bracket and arch wire.

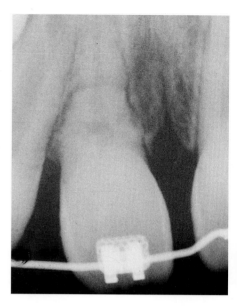

Fig. 5.28 Radiograph of 11 (same patient as in Figs 5.26, 5.27) one year later at initiation of active orthodontic treatment.

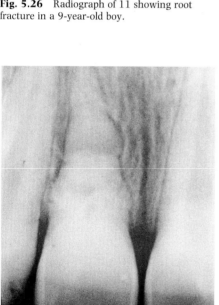

Fig. 5.29 Radiograph of 11 (same patient) five years after original injury showing successful outcome.

tissue, orthodontic movement may again cause further separation of the fragments or, in intrusive movement, unpredictable resorption. A root fractured tooth with Type II healing is, in fact, a short rooted tooth and may be treated as such. In essence, orthodontic movement of root fractured teeth should be carried out with caution but should not be a contra-indication to such treatment. It might be suggested, in these days of adhesive bridges and single tooth implants, that even should orthodontic treatment hasten the loss of a root fractured tooth, this is not such a disaster if it means that the final arrangement of the teeth is overall to the advantage of the patient and his/her dentition.

FURTHER READING

Andreasen, F. M. and Andreasen, J. O. (1988). Resorption and mineralisation processes following root fracture of permanent incisors. *Endodontics and Dental Traumatology*, **4**, 202–14.

Andreasen, J. O. (1981). *Traumatic injuries of the teeth*, (2nd edn). Munksgaard, Copenhagen.

Andreasen, F. M., Andreasen, J. O., and Bayer, T. (1989). Prognosis of root-fractured permanent incisors—prediction of healing modalities. *Endodontics and Dental Traumatology*, **5**, 11–22.

Jacobsen, I (1976). Root fracture in permanent anterior teeth with incomplete root formation. *Scandinavian Journal of Dental Research*, **84**, 210–17.

Zachrisson, B. U. and Jacobsen, I. (1975). Long-term prognosis of 66 permanent anterior teeth with root fracture. *Scandinavian Journal of Dental Research*, **83**, 345–54.

6 Luxation injuries

6　Luxation injuries

Luxation injuries account for between 15 and 60% of oro-dental injuries in the permanent dentition. The wide range can be accounted for, in part, by the fact that the less severe forms of luxation injury leave no lasting sign and are, therefore, overlooked or not identified in epidemiological studies.

Five types of luxation injury are described, together with avulsion (total luxation), where the tooth is knocked out completely:

Concussion	No abnormal loosening or displacement, but marked reaction to percussion.
Subluxation (loosening)	Abnormal loosening, but no clinical or radiographic displacement.
Lateral luxation	Displacement of tooth other than in its long axis.
Intrusive luxation	Displacement of tooth apically, into the alveolar bone.
Extrusive luxation	Displacement of tooth coronally, partially out of its socket.
Total luxation (avulsion)	Displacement of tooth coronally, completely out of its socket.

Each type of luxation injury will be considered, and its management described, separately.

CONCUSSION

Concussion is a minor injury with minimal damage to the tooth and periodontal tissues. The tooth is of normal colour with no detectable hard tissue damage and is firm in its socket. It is not displaced but exhibits an exaggerated response to gentle percussion, probably because of some bleeding and associated oedema in the periodontal ligament (Fig. 6.1). However, as the damage to the periodontal ligament is slight, there is no bleeding at the gingival margin.

Vitality testing

A positive response to routine thermal and electrical vitality tests may be expected, confirming that there has been little or no damage to the neurovascular supply to the tooth. Nevertheless, a small proportion do not respond immediately following the injury but recover within a week or so.

Radiographs

It is usual to take a periapical radiograph to ensure that other damage is not overlooked, to assess the state of root development and tooth maturity and to serve as a 'baseline' for follow-up care.

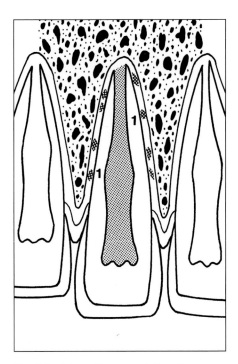

Fig. 6.1 Schematic representation of concussion. Damage to the periodontal ligament (1) results in an exaggerated response to percussion.

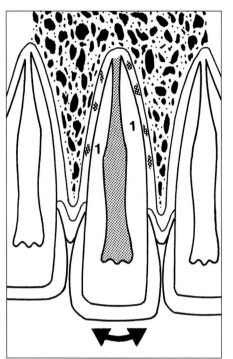

Fig. 6.2 Schematic representation of subluxation. Damage to the periodontal ligament (1) with associated gingival bleeding and mobility of the tooth (arrow) are diagnostic features.

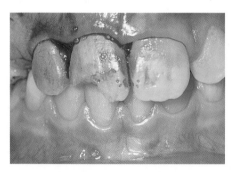

Fig. 6.3 Subluxed 12, 11. Note bleeding at gingival margin.

Treatment

Treatment is usually limited to reassurance and advice to avoid biting directly on to the damaged tooth and the maintenance of a soft diet for a few days. Simple analgesics, such as paracetamol, may also be recommended. Occasionally, it may be necessary to relieve occlusion with the opposing teeth by selective grinding—this is more likely in older patients where the dentition is mature.

Follow-up

As with all teeth that have been injured, the damaged tooth should be reviewed after one month, three months, six months, and then at the patient's regular dental check-up visits. There is a risk of loss of vitality, albeit small (approximately 3%), almost invariably confined to mature teeth.

About 5% of teeth affected by concussion have been shown to develop an apical radiolucency and superficial root resorption, a condition known as 'transient apical breakdown'. A similiar proportion are affected by pulpal obliteration which begins in the coronal pulp and progresses apically over some months or even years. However, intervention is not necessary as resolution of any apical radiolucency and spontaneous cessation of the resorption is the norm. The pulpal obliteration has often been described as 'nature's own root filling' and although the late development of necrosis and infection in the thin thread of residual pulp tissue in the sclerosed canal has been reported, this is considered to be less common than complications arising from the endodontic therapy that would be necessary to treat it.

SUBLUXATION (LOOSENING)

Subluxation (Fig. 6.2) is also a relatively minor injury in which the hard tissues of the teeth are spared but there is damage to the periodontal tissues with tearing of some of the ligament fibres, bleeding, and oedema. The tooth, which is not displaced, is of normal colour but there is bleeding at the gingival margin and, when gently palpated or percussed, it is tender and exhibits abnormal mobility (Fig. 6.3).

Vitality testing

Approximately 55% of subluxed teeth do not respond to vitality tests in the first few days after the injury but most, especially the less mature, recover within about four weeks.

Radiographs

As with concussion, a radiograph is taken to ensure that there is no other damage and to assess the state of root development and tooth maturity and to serve as the 'baseline' for follow-up care.

Treatment

Having reassured the patient and parent as to the limited extent of the injury, it is sometimes necessary to relieve occlusal interferences caused by extrusion of the tooth because of oedema in the damaged periodontal ligament. Most subluxed teeth rapidly become firm again without active treatment. Splinting such teeth is only rarely indicated and is then usually done to increase the patient's comfort and confidence, as there is little evidence that it improves healing. A soft diet and simple analgesics, such as paracetamol, may be recommended until any discomfort has subsided.

Follow-up

The damaged tooth should be reviewed in the same way as already described for concussed teeth. The risk of loss of vitality is somewhat greater—approximately 12%—and as with concussion, almost invariably affects mature teeth.

Transient apical breakdown may be seen in about 4% of subluxed teeth, pulpal obliteration in about 10%, and a few show apical radiolucency. Although this is a more severe injury when compared with concussion, the risk of complications is only slightly greater and, therefore, a satisfactory outcome is generally to be expected.

LATERAL LUXATION

In lateral luxation, the crown of the tooth is usually displaced palatally (Fig. 6.4) or labially but the displacement may also have a mesial or distal component. With palatal displacements, the apex moves buccally as the crown moves palatally and there is a tendency in the more severe cases for the root apex to perforate the buccal plate (Fig. 6.4, 5). In some instances the tooth moves bodily in a labial as well as apical direction, fracturing the buccal plate which may then be displaced with it (Fig. 6.4, 2). In labial displacements the apex tends to stay in its original position while the crown is tilted labially, either breaking through the buccal plate or carrying the buccal plate with it.

Palatal displacement of the crown will frequently result in interference with the opposing teeth when the patient closes his/her teeth together (Fig. 6.5). Following the injury, the tooth may be firm in its displaced position or it may be mobile.

Vitality testing

Routine thermal and electrical vitality testing will often produce no response because of the disruption to the apical neurovascular bundle. In the less common labial displacement this disruption is less severe than that resulting from palatal displacement, avulsion, intrusive, or extrusive luxation, where much apical movement results. In many cases, a positive response will return within a few weeks, particularly if the apex has not moved so far as to tear the apical vessels or, again, in the younger patient with an immature tooth where there is good reparative potential.

Radiographs

A periapical radiograph is taken of the affected tooth, to ensure that other damage is not overlooked, to assess the state of root development and tooth maturity, and to serve as a 'baseline' for follow-up care. As laterally luxated teeth may also suffer root fracture, especially in older patients with mature teeth, it is recommended that a standard occlusal view is taken in addition to the regular periapical view.

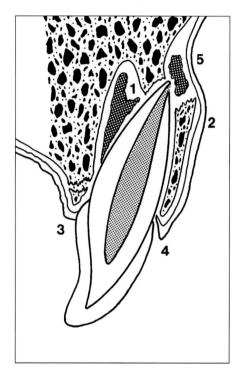

Fig. 6.4 Schematic representation of a lateral luxation. In more severe cases the apex escapes from the confines of the socket (1) and becomes locked (5). The alveolar crest palatally may be fractured (3) and there is bleeding at the gingival margin (4).

Treatment

There are three main clinical presentations in lateral luxation (in the absence of other damage) and the clinical management of each type is considered separately:

1. Tooth mobile

The tooth should be gently repositioned with digital pressure, aligning it as accurately as possible and ensuring that no occlusal interference results. It should then be splinted for 7–10 days which will allow soft tissue healing. After 7–10 days, the splint is removed to assess the degree of stabilization—it is advisable to return the tooth to normal function as soon as possible as this reduces the tendency for ankylosis to develop during healing. However, a further period of splinting may be necessary if the tooth is still very loose, perhaps because of fracture of part of the alveolar process—a feature more often seen in older patients.

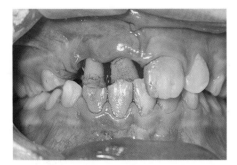

Fig. 6.5 Laterally luxated 12, 11. The crowns of these teeth are firmly locked in a palatal position and are in reverse overjet with the lower teeth.

2. Tooth firm, with occlusal interference (Fig. 6.5)

The ideal management of laterally luxated teeth which are firm in their displaced position and interfere with the opposing teeth has yet to be shown conclusively. Some authorities recommend immediate surgical realignment of the tooth while others suggest that this may cause further root surface damage and advise that the realignment should be carried out orthodontically. The choice of method will depend to some extent on the co-operation of the patient and to some extent on the degree of displacement. For example, if the tooth apex has perforated the buccal plate (Fig. 6.4, 5) surgical repositioning may be advisable so that the apex may be disengaged from its locked buccal position.

Immediate realignment under local analgesia

The thumb is placed buccally over the root apex and the forefinger hooked behind the crown incisally and with a firm squeeze, the crown is moved labially as the root is pressed back into its socket. When the apex has perforated the buccal plate, pressure with the thumb will have to be exerted in such a way that the apex disengages from its locked position and allows the tooth to spring back into its original position. It will now be quite mobile and should, therefore, be splinted. Ideally, splinting should be for 7–10 days while preliminary healing takes place. This enables the tooth to return to function as soon as possible and reduces the change of ankylosis. However, as already mentioned in (1), if the tooth is still very loose (perhaps because of fracture of part of the alveolar process) a further period of splinting may be required.

Orthodontic realignment

An alginate impression is taken, a simple removable appliance made and fitted within 24 hours. The appliance should have cribs for retention, posterior capping to disengage the occlusal interference, and a spring (T-, or recurved) which is activated to realign the displaced tooth, usually after two–three weeks when preliminary healing is well under way.

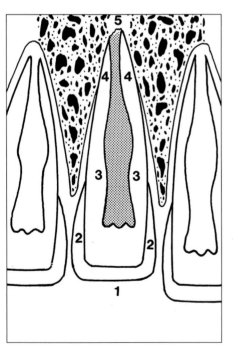

Fig. 6.6 Schematic representation of intrusive luxation. The periodontal ligament space is lost (4) and there is malalignment relative to the adjacent teeth (1, 2). Pulp necrosis (3) is expected in all mature teeth and at least 60% of immature teeth.

3. Tooth firm but no occlusal interference

When the displaced tooth is firm but does not interfere with the opposing teeth on closure there are again two ways in which the problem may be dealt with. To date, on the basis of available evidence, neither method shows an advantage over the other in terms of clinical outcome. Some authorities recommend immediate surgical realignment of the tooth, as described in (2). On the other hand, others suggest that this may cause further root surface damage and advise that the tooth is left in its displaced position when it will either realign naturally under the influence of normal soft tissue activity, or may be realigned orthodontically. The choice of method will again be influenced both by the co-operation of the patient and the extent of the displacement.

INTRUSIVE LUXATION

In intrusive luxation, the tooth is displaced apically with little or no deflection (Fig. 6.6). Occasionally, the root of the tooth may perforate the floor of the nose. Coronal fractures can be superimposed on the displacement injury but root fractures are extremely rare.

Prompt assessment is particularly important with intrusive luxation—inadequate care and treatment in the early stages significantly reduces the prognosis for the intruded tooth. Even apparently quite trivial degrees of intrusion can result in unexpectedly severe complications.

Diagnosis

The diagnosis of an intruded tooth is often straightforward (Fig. 6.7). This is particularly the case in older patients whose dentition is stable, as the tooth in question is readily seen to be in a more apical position than the neighbouring teeth. In addition, the patient will often say that 'the tooth has been pushed up into the gum'.

In the younger patient, however, the situation is frequently less clear. Permanent teeth do not erupt at exactly the same time nor at the same rate, left versus right. An intruded tooth may, in such circumstances, be overlooked. Gentle percussion of an intruded tooth elicits essentially the same percussive note as an ankylosed tooth—a high pitched 'cracked cup' or metallic sound. It is recommended, therefore, that during the clinical examination of any patient with a history of injury to their permanent front teeth, all teeth in the area are gently percussed. Intruded teeth are then less likely to be overlooked.

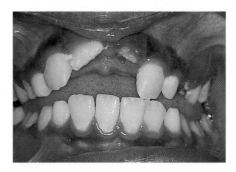

Fig. 6.7 Intrusive luxation of 11, 21.

Vitality testing

Most intruded teeth do not respond to routine vitality testing initially and as the majority become non-vital (see below) regaining a response to such testing is very much the exception rather than the rule.

Radiographs

Routine intra-oral films of the area of the injury usually suffice unless the degree of apical displacement is so severe that it is unclear where the tooth is lying. In that case, a lateral view or a lateral skull view may help to determine the tooth's position. Sometimes, on first examination it is thought that the tooth has been knocked right out until it is revealed on the radiographs to be present but considerably displaced. A significant radiographic feature of an intruded tooth is the loss of the periodontal ligament space particularly in the more apical portion of the root (Fig. 6.8).

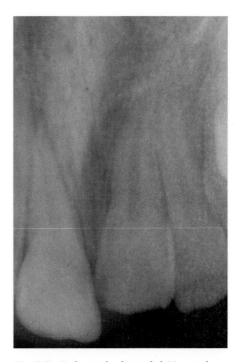

Fig. 6.8 Radiograph of intruded 21: note loss of periodontal ligament space in the more apical portion of the root.

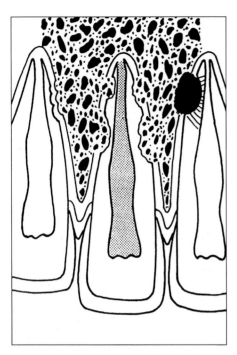

Fig. 6.9 Schematic representation of the three main types of external root resorption (left to right): surface resorption; replacement resorption; inflammatory resorption.

Tissue responses to intrusive luxation

An intrusive luxation is a violent displacement of the tooth in its socket with significant movement of the tooth in its long axis. The immediate consequences of this are:

(1) the crushing and rupture of many of the periodontal ligament fibres;
(2) the crushing of some areas of cementum, and the loss of other areas torn from the root surface;
(3) the crushing of the neurovascular tissues supplying the pulp (and the pulp tissue itself in immature teeth).

The *complications* which may arise from these tissue effects are:

(a) loss of pulp vitality;
(b) surface root resorption (self-limiting);
(c) external *replacement* root resorption (usually slow), with associated ankylosis;
(d) external *inflammatory* root resorption (very rapid).

All intruded *mature* teeth lose vitality, as do at least 60% of *immature* teeth. At first it seems surprising that many immature teeth, with their excellent blood supply and considerable reparative potential, should fair little better than mature teeth. The probable explanation is that because of the wide apical foramen the pulp tissue is subjected to significant crush injury as the tooth moves apically. In the mature tooth the apical blood vessels are torn and crushed, severing the pulp's neurovascular supply.

Intruded *immature teeth* have the potential for re-eruption but *mature teeth* do not.

External root resorption

Root resorption may be physiological as, for example, during replacement of deciduous teeth by their permanent successors, or pathological. External root resorption as a response to injury will be considered to be pathological in many cases because although it is often associated with healing, its effects are frequently found to be deleterious (Fig. 6.9).

Surface root resorption

This is usually a fairly trivial response to intrusive luxation (and other forms of injury involving axial movement of the tooth). It is characterized by resorption of small areas of cementum and dentine which resolves spontaneously. These small areas are sometimes evident radiographically as an irregularity of the root surface.

External replacement root resorption

This is the relatively slow replacement of the root dentine by bone (which produces an ankylosis) and develops following the loss of root surface cementum (Fig. 6.10). This loss of cementum may be the consequence of violent, vertical movement of the tooth within the socket when pieces of cementum are pulled off the root surface, or the cementum is crushed and becomes necrotic (intrusion, extrusion, and avulsion), or it becomes necrotic because the root surface has been allowed to dry out prior to replantation following avulsion. As healing takes place, the necrotic cementum is removed or resorbed by the body's natural defence mechanisms. This loss of the cementum layer on the root surface seems

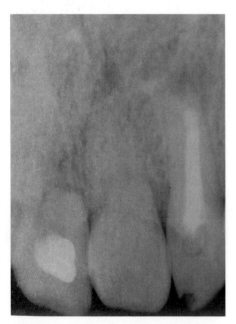

Fig. 6.10 External replacement resorption affecting 21, replanted two years previously.

to expose the dentine to resorptive attack and its replacement by bone which although slow is usually progressive and leads, eventually, to loss of the tooth. It is as if the tooth is no longer recognized as 'self' and is, therefore, rejected by the body.

External inflammatory root resorption

This is usually characterized by an extremely rapid loss of areas of the root dentine (Fig. 6.11). The rapidity can be such that in an affected area the whole thickness of the dentine may be resorbed from the root surface through to the pulp chamber within 4–5 weeks. Several areas of resorptive attack are seen radiographically as radiolucent areas on the root surface and involving the immediately adjacent bone (Fig. 6.12). Again, one of the triggers for the initiation of the resorption is loss of cementum from the root surface as previously described, but an additional factor which encourages the aggressive resorptive process is the presence of an infected necrotic pulp. Bacteria migrate from the pulp chamber along the dentinal tubules towards the root surface. Where the cementum has been lost, bacterial metabolites have a direct effect on the tissues at the root surface encouraging osteoclastic activity, which is sustained by the lowered pH associated with the inflammatory process, and results in resorption at these 'denuded' root surface sites.

In both major types of external root resorption, the necrotic pulp should be removed and, following thorough mechanical cleansing and irrigation, the root canal should be obturated with a non-setting calcium hydroxide medicament. This will kill bacteria in the root canal and, particularly, those in the dentinal tubules. It is also thought that the high alkalinity of calcium hydroxide will raise the pH at the root surface, discouraging the osteoclastic activity responsible for the resorption. In immature teeth, apical barrier formation will also result, enabling the satisfactory placement of a conventional root filling later.

Treatment

In many cases, the result of intrusive luxation is pulp necrosis and infection. The objective of treatment, therefore, is to reposition the intruded tooth so that endodontic therapy with calcium hydroxide can be instituted within 3–4 weeks, before infection of the non-vital pulp and/or either major type of external root resorption can become established.

Repositioning the tooth may be carried out surgically, the repositioned tooth being splinted in its corrected position for 7–10 days. Short splinting periods are preferable to longer ones as the tendency for ankylosis developing during the healing process is much reduced when the tooth is brought back into function as quickly as possible. Nevertheless, significant external root resorption is a very common sequel in this type of injury, although there are, as yet, few studies on the effectiveness of the early institution of endodontic therapy with calcium hydroxide in these cases.

Repositioning may also be achieved over 3–4 weeks using orthodontic techniques which are thought by some to offer a less traumatic alternative. The forces used are essentially physiological and the root surface is not exposed to the risk of further physical damage which may result from handling or drying out, albeit for short periods, during the surgery.

Once the tooth has been extruded sufficiently for access to be made to the pulp chamber endodontic therapy is started. Following removal of the necrotic pulp, estimation of the working length, thorough mechanical cleansing, irrigation, and drying, the canal is obturated with a non-setting calcium hydroxide paste and

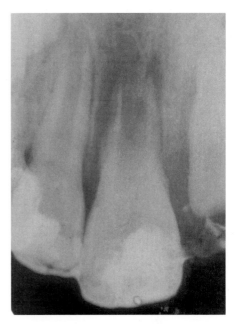

Fig. 6.11 External inflammatory root resorption (early) affecting non-vital 11, replanted three months previously.

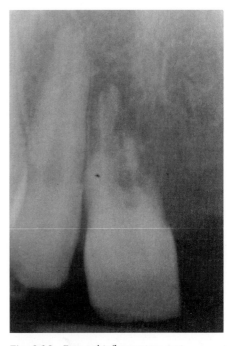

Fig. 6.12 External inflammatory root resorption (advanced) affecting 11, 8 months post-replantation. The tooth had been stored in milk for 4 hours, replanted but received no follow-up endodontic care.

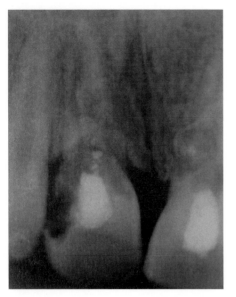

Fig. 6.13 External replacement root resorption (advanced) affecting 11, 21, five years post-replantation. The teeth had dried out but were replanted. Endodontic treatment has failed to arrest the resorption.

the access cavity sealed with a suitable cement (e.g. polycarboxylate). One month later the patient is recalled and in the absence of adverse signs or symptoms the dressing is removed, the calcium hydroxide washed out of the canal and the canal dried and filled, as before, with calcium hydroxide. The calcium hydroxide should be replaced every 6–8 months. A definitive root filling should be placed once it has become apparent that the treatment has been successful and, in the case of immature teeth, apical repair and hard tissue barrier formation has taken place. If the treatment has been unsuccessful and external inflammatory root resorption has resulted in extensive loss of tissue the tooth will usually have to be extracted. In some cases, however, the failed treatment may have resulted in the development of slowly progressing replacement resorption when the tooth may survive for several years before it finally loses all root support (Fig. 6.13), and has to be extracted and a prosthetic replacement provided.

EXTRUSIVE LUXATION

In extrusive luxation (Fig. 6.14) the tooth is displaced partly out of the socket in a coronal direction. In principle, the management of such a tooth differs little from that for a totally luxated (avulsed) tooth, which is described in detail in the next section. In essence, however, once clinical (Fig. 6.15) and radiographic examination (Fig. 6.16) have confirmed the diagnosis and excluded other injury, the tooth should be repositioned using firm digital pressure and splinted for 7–10 days. Local analgesia will frequently not be required and the associated vasoconstrictive effects of most local analgesic solutions may, in fact, be a disadvantage.

Regular follow-up is necessary so that should the pulp become necrotic, endodontic therapy may be instituted to intercept the deleterious effects of its subsequent infection.

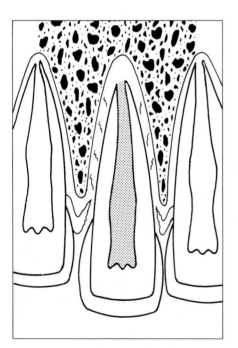

Fig. 6.14 Schematic representation of extrusive luxation.

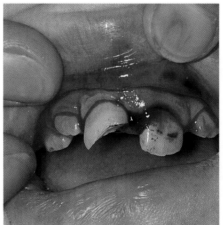

Fig. 6.15 Extruded 21; fracture of 11 involving enamel and dentine.

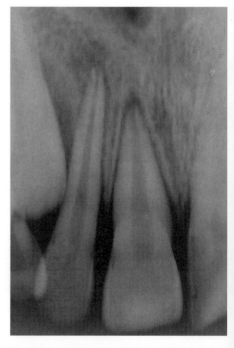

Fig. 6.16 Radiograph of 11, showing the typical widening of the periodontal ligament space associated with extrusive luxation.

TOTAL LUXATION (AVULSION)

Avulsion (total luxation) (Fig. 6.17) is a rare injury. However, perhaps more than in many other types of injury, the promptness with which appropriate treatment is instituted will have a direct bearing on the outcome.

The ideal treatment for an avulsed tooth (Figs 6.18, 6.19) is its immediate replacement in the socket (Fig. 6.20).

The first contact may be a telephone call from a local school or the parent or friend of a child who has knocked out a front tooth, when the advice will usually be to replace the tooth in its socket straight away. If the tooth is dirty, it may be rinsed under running tap water (but should not be scrubbed!) to remove loose debris. Although tap water is potentially damaging because it is not isotonic, any harmful effect is considerably outweighed by the advantage of having the tooth back in the socket as quickly as possible where the remaining water is rapidly replaced by isotonic tissue fluid.

If the tooth cannot be replaced straight away, the patient should be brought to the surgery as soon as possible bringing the tooth with them in a suitable transport medium (e.g. milk). Other suitable transport media include normal saline and contact lens fluid. The medium should be physiological to minimize further damage to the periodontal ligament and, most particularly, the root surface cementum since necrosis of the cementum can lead to the development of replacement resorption and concommitant ankylosis.

At the surgery

If the tooth has not been replanted, it should be placed in sterile normal saline. The history is taken and if soil contamination of any wound is a possibility the patient's tetanus immunization state should also be checked so that a booster can be arranged later if necessary. A clinical examination is carried out and a radiograph of the empty socket taken to ensure that the alveolar bone is intact. However, as time is of the essence in the care of this type of injury, vitality testing of adjacent teeth, which may also have been damaged, and further radiographic examination are usually delayed until the avulsed tooth has been dealt with.

Replant or not?

The decision now has to be taken as to whether the tooth should be replanted, or not. In most cases replacing the tooth in its socket will be appropriate. Nevertheless, there will be some occasions when replantation is not the best treatment. This can often be difficult to explain to parents who have become

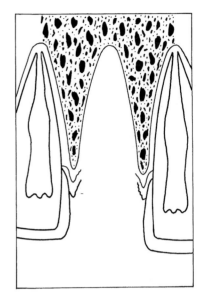

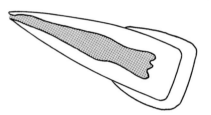

Fig. 6.17 Schematic representation of total luxation (avulsion).

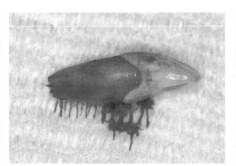

Fig. 6.18 Avulsed 11.

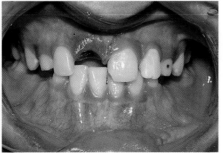

Fig. 6.19 11 was knocked out 20 minutes previously.

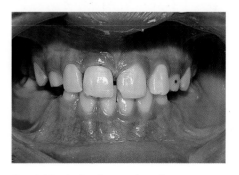

Fig. 6.20 11 has been replanted.

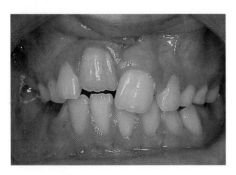

Fig. 6.21 Upper right central incisor (11) had been out of the socket for five hours, stored dry, before replantation two years ago. Ankylosis has resulted in the replanted tooth being left behind as the other teeth have continued to erupt.

accustomed to the idea that teeth can be put back in when they have been knocked out.

A tooth which has been inadequately stored prior to replantation, particularly when allowed to dry out, will invariably begin to undergo external replacement root resorption, with associated ankylosis following replantation. The presence of a non-vital pulp which will usually be infected, may also give rise to external inflammatory root resorption, which in turn will lead to rapid loss of much of the root. Both forms of external root resorption may be slowed down or arrested by endodontic treatment with a calcium hydroxide medicament, although the ankylosis associated with replacement resorption will usually persist.

The development of an ankylosis in a young patient in whom there will still be significant growth of the alveolus results in the replanted tooth being left behind as the other teeth continue to erupt (Fig. 6.21). The resulting discrepancy in the alveolar contour can be very difficult to manage, especially when the alveolus fails to remodel satisfactorily after the tooth has had to be removed. The defect in hard tissue is frequently difficult to disguise particularly when the patient has a high lip line.

In the older patient, in whom all or most of the alveolar growth has taken place, the development of ankylosis is much less of a problem and is, therefore, not a contra-indication to replantation in this age group.

Technique of replantation

Any dirt is carefully rinsed off the root of the tooth, taking care not to damage the ligament or cementum and as endodontic therapy is often required later, the length of the tooth is recorded. The tooth is then pushed firmly up into socket—local analgesia is frequently not needed. There is, presently, some debate as to whether the blood clot should be rinsed from the socket, or not, prior to replantation. Until recently, it has been accepted that up to 48 hours after avulsion, the blood clot is satisfactorily displaced as the tooth is pressed into the socket during replantation. However, there has been a suggestion that the presence of blood clot between the root surface and the socket wall may encourage external root resorption. Further studies are required before a definitive answer to this problem can be given. The authors suggest that if the patient's co-operation allows, the blood clot should be removed by gently irrigating the socket with sterile normal saline prior to replanting the tooth. If such an additional procedure might compromise the patient's co-operation and, therefore, the replantation, then it is acceptable to replace the tooth without removing the blood clot first.

In some cases difficulty may be experienced in replanting the tooth because of damage to the socket wall. While it may be possible to reposition the displaced bony fragment(s) and then replant the tooth, it should be noted that the chances of a successful outcome will be reduced.

Splinting

The replanted tooth is splinted for 7–10 days. Longer periods of splinting encourage ankylosis. Usually, the most practical form of splint will be that fabricated from a short piece of stainless steel wire held onto the replanted tooth and its firmer neighbours with acid-etch-retained composite (Fig. 6.22).

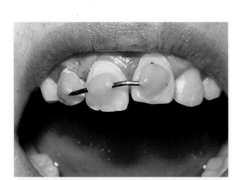

Fig. 6.22 Simple splint of stainless steel wire attached to the teeth by acid-etch-retained composite supporting replanted 11.

Antibiotics

A five-day course of antibiotics is prescribed to cover the immediate post-replantation period. Penicillin is the drug of choice with erythromycin as a suitable alternative for those who are allergic to the penicillins. The dose is adjusted to suit the age and weight of the patient.

Tooth maturity

Immature teeth which have been appropriately stored may be expected to revascularize if replanted within two hours of their avulsion.

Mature teeth, however, and inappropriately stored immature teeth do not revascularize. An essential aspect of their management, therefore, will be root canal therapy which is instituted at the end of the splinting period (Fig. 6.23). This involves the usual thorough mechanical cleansing of the root canal to remove necrotic pulp tissue and infected dentine, irrigation with sodium hypochlorite solution, and obturation of the root canal with a non-setting calcium hydroxide paste (Fig. 6.24). The calcium hydroxide paste should be replenished after one month and then every six to eight months until a permanent root filling is placed (Fig. 6.25).

The calcium hydroxide controls or prevents the development of bacterial infection within the root canal and probably raises the pH at the root surface in those areas where pieces of cementum have been lost. This will discourage or prevent external root resorption in mature and immature teeth. In addition, in immature teeth, an apical barrier will form, facilitating the subsequent placement of a permanent root filling.

However, in *immature teeth*, it is recommended that placement of the permanent root filling is delayed until any orthodontic tooth movement has been completed. This is because of a tendency for the calcific barrier to be resorbed during orthodontic tooth movement which can result in breakdown of the apical seal and lead to premature failure of the root filling.

In *mature teeth*, a permanent root filling is not placed until at least *one year* after replantation.

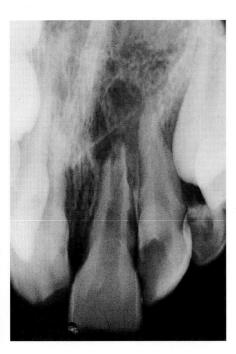

Fig. 6.23 Replanted, immature 21 which has not revascularized (evidence of infection and early inflammatory resorption).

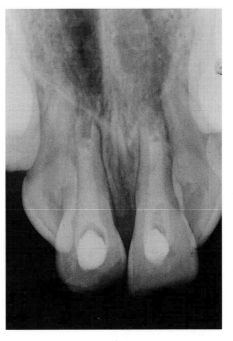

Fig. 6.24 Calcium hydroxide obturating the root canals of 11 and 21 (same patient as in Fig. 6.23).

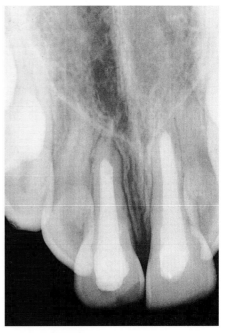

Fig. 6.25 Completed root fillings in 11 and 21 (same patient as in Figs 6.23, 6.24).

As has already been indicated, the *main complications* associated with replantation of avulsed teeth are:

1. Pulp necrosis and infection which may lead to the development of external inflammatory root resorption. This type of external root resorption is extremely rapid and much of the root can be lost within a few months of the replantation if steps are not taken to prevent or control it.

2. External replacement root resorption consequent on necrosis of the periodontal ligament and cementum. This type of external root resorption is usually slow but in the younger patient the associated ankylosis tends to result in unsightly infra-occlusion of the replanted tooth (Fig. 6.21). The aesthetic management of this problem can be very difficult.

FURTHER READING

Anderson, L. and Bodin, I. (1990). Avulsed human teeth replanted within 15 minutes—a long-term clinical follow-up study. *Endodontics and Dental Traumatology*, **6**, 37–42.

Andreasen, J. O. and Andreasen, F. M. (1994). *Textbook and color atlas of traumatic injuries to the teeth*, (3rd edn). Munksgaard, Copenhagen.

7 Non-vital immature teeth: late presentation

7   Non-vital immature teeth: late presentation

The non-vital immature permanent tooth is frequently a late presentation of oro-dental injury. An exception is that resulting from the presence of an invaginated odontome (*dens in dente*) which has caused pulp necrosis. Careful questioning of the patient or parent, only rarely elicits a clear history of trauma, although many patients provide a vague report of the tooth having had a 'slight bump' some time ago. A small proportion of injured teeth which have been regularly monitored following an accident lose, or fail to regain, their vitality. It is often difficult to decide exactly when the tooth has become non-vital as equivocal results are often obtained when applying conventional pulp vitality tests following trauma. In the absence of signs or symptoms of infection arising from a necrotic pulp, it is sensible to wait at least three months following oro-dental injury before deciding that a tooth has lost, or failed to regain, its vitality. In some cases, a response to routine vitality testing may take more than a year to return.

CLINICAL PRESENTATION

The non-vital immature permanent tooth may present in a number of ways:

- a painless, sometimes discoloured tooth with an associated 'gum boil' or draining sinus, perhaps of several months duration—it may be firm or mobile;
- a painful, mobile, tooth with associated soft tissue swelling;
- a coincidental finding when the patient is being assessed for another problem such as malocclusion or even trauma to an adjacent tooth—it may be revealed during clinical examination or as a chance finding on a radiograph.
- during the follow-up of an injured tooth, particularly after luxation injury, when it becomes apparent from clinical and radiographic evidence that the pulp has become necrotic.

The diagnosis of pulp necrosis is based on clinical signs (e.g. discolouration, mobility, presence of a sinus, etc.), the absence of response to thermal or electrical vitality testing, the radiographic appearance of the immature tooth, often with associated signs of loss of lamina dura and/or an apical radiolucency (Figs 7.1, 7.2).

The non-vital tooth is almost always infected, usually with a mixed population of oral commensals. The source of these organisms is unclear but the majority probably originate from the bloodstream or the gingival crevice. The clinical management involves conventional endodontic techniques—adequate mechanical debridement of the canal and the use of an irrigant known to dissolve organic debris (e.g. sodium hypochlorite), followed by obturation of the root canal with a medicament that will kill any remaining microorganisms.

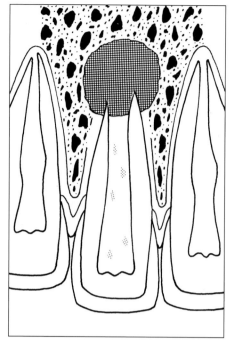

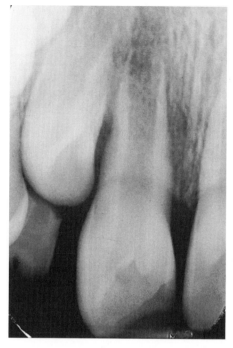

Fig. 7.1 Schematic representation of non-vital immature permanent upper incisor tooth with apical infection and periapical bone loss.

Fig. 7.2 Radiograph of 11 which is non-vital, immature and shows periapical infection and bone loss.

The walls of the root canal of an immature tooth, especially in the apical region, are thin. Endodontic preparation, therefore, has to be carried out with care to ensure that damage is not caused by over-zealous instrumentation.

Root canal therapy in immature permanent incisor teeth invariably leaves the tooth further weakened by the large access cavity required to enable thorough preparation of the canal, particularly when the apical region is divergent. If the tooth is discoloured it may not be possible to restore it with a jacket crown. However, composite or porcelain veneers, attached to the labial enamel after etching, frequently provide a very satisfactory solution to the problem.

CLINICAL MANAGEMENT

Although many non-vital immature teeth are symptomless, the initial presentation can be one of acute infection, sometimes with an associated facial swelling and systemic disturbance.

In these cases, the acute infection should be brought under control by establishing drainage via an access cavity into the pulp chamber. Any solid pieces of necrotic pulp tissue should be removed with a barbed broach and the canal irrigated with hypochlorite solution (1% w/v). Ideally, the canal should then be further debrided with a large (size 50–80) Hedstrom file, irrigated, dried, a dressing placed (polyantibiotic paste or antiseptic or calcium hydroxide—see below), and the access cavity sealed. If the infection is particularly severe, or the child too distressed, it may be necessary to leave the tooth on open drainage. This should be for no more than 24 hours. Systemic antibiotics may also be prescribed. However, as a general principle antibiotics should only be prescribed once adequate drainage has been obtained. It is poor clinical practice to use systemic antibiotics alone to control infection originating from a necrotic, infected pulp, although there may be occasions when the clinician has no choice, perhaps because of poor patient compliance when first seen.

More usually, the presentation of this clinical problem is that of a chronically infected tooth. In all cases the clinical management, once any acute infection has been brought under control, follows a similar course. The technique described by Cvek (1972), itself the development of the methods of earlier workers, is recommended. In essence, a calcium hydroxide slurry or paste is used to obturate the root canal of the immature tooth after thorough mechanical cleansing. Calcium hydroxide has a high pH (approximately 11) and is, therefore, bactericidal. Resolution of the infection may then be expected, followed by healing in the periapical tissues and the development of a hard tissue barrier across the apical foramen of the immature tooth, against which a conventional root filling may subsequently be condensed. This apical repair and barrier formation has been shown to take place within as little as two months, although at that stage the barrier is not particularly robust. Generally, the barrier will be sufficiently well formed for placement of a conventional root filling within six months although in some cases it may take as long as 18 months. After that time it must be assumed that little further repair will take place.

Fig. 7.3 Palatal aspect of 21 showing the large access cavity necessary for endodontic therapy in immature permanent incisor teeth.

Clinical technique

1. Isolate the tooth.
2. Gain access to the pulp chamber via the cingulum and adjust the access cavity so that it incorporates most of the coronal pulp and it is possible to have a straight line access to the more apical parts of the canal. The access cavity in immature permanent teeth is, of necessity, large taking up to one-third of the width of the crown (Fig. 7.3). It is also important to remember that the long axis of the crown of the tooth and that of the root are not co-incident, the root is angled palatally with respect to the crown. If the labial surface of the crown of the tooth is used as a guide when preparing the access cavity, there is a real danger that the root canal could be perforated labially, several millimetres below the gingival margin. When preparing the access cavity, therefore, it is often necessary to remove dentine from the palatal aspect of the crown–root canal junction. Rarely, it may be necessary to gain access via a labial approach—when, for example, the crown of the tooth is particularly recurved so that it is not possible to have a straight access to the more apical parts of the canal by the more usual access.
3. Establish the length of the root by taking a radiograph with an endodontic instrument of known length in the canal (Fig. 7.4). The working length should be 1 mm short of the radiographic apex to avoid damage to any viable cells in this region (perhaps remnants of Hertwig's root sheath), which could produce new dentine.
4. File the canal to remove necrotic pulp remnants and infected debris using a large Hedstrom file (e.g. size 60, which is quite thick while retaining some flexibility).
5. Using a small hypodermic syringe and needle thoroughly irrigate the canal with hypochlorite solution (1% w/v), allowing the solution to remain in the canal for 30 seconds at a time to assist in dislodging the organic debris, followed by sterile physiological saline. When no more debris is being displaced, draw off the fluid remaining in the root canal with the syringe and discard it and dry the root canal using large paper points.
6. Fill the canal with a non-setting calcium hydroxide paste. Use either a proprietary preparation or a paste made by mixing calcium hydroxide powder with sterile water or saline. It may be encouraged into the apical part of the canal by the careful use of a spiral root canal filler.

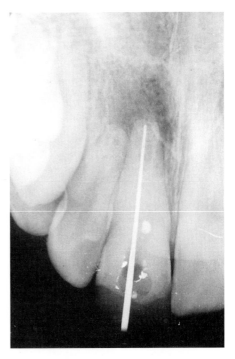

Fig. 7.4 Diagnostic radiograph with instrument of known length in the root canal.

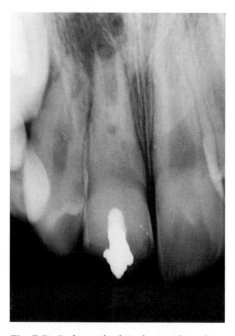

Fig. 7.5 Radiograph of 11 showing loss of calcium hydroxide from the apical portion of the root canal some months after placement.

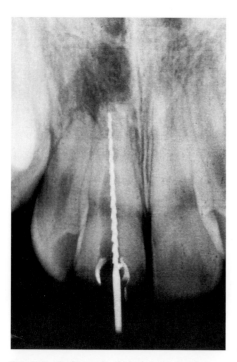

Fig. 7.6 Radiograph of 11 showing hard tissue barrier at the apex and endodontic instrument within the root canal against the barrier.

7. Gently compress the calcium hydroxide in the canal using a small cotton pledget and leave a small cotton pledget in the pulp chamber.

8. Seal the access cavity with a temporary cement. Avoid cements containing eugenol as these tend to discolour the crown of the tooth and particularly any overlying composite material used to restore the tooth. Polycarboxylate or zinc phosphate cements are suitable. Take a radiograph to ensure that the calcium hydroxide has successfully occluded the lumen of the root canal—if not repeat stages 5–8.

9. Arrange to review the patient after three months.

At the review appointment, examine the patient to ensure that there is no overt infection, take a radiograph to determine the degree of resolution of the apical infection and to ensure that the calcium hydroxide still occludes the root canal and, all being well, arrange a further review after another six months. If the calcium hydroxide has partially or totally resorbed (Fig. 7.5) it should be replenished before arranging the review.

At the next review, the usual clinical examination is carried out and if there are no clinical signs of infection, proceed to the next stage which involves removing the dressing from the canal and testing for the formation of an apical barrier:

(a) isolate the tooth;

(b) remove the dressing from the access cavity, remove the cotton pledget and wash out the calcium hydroxide paste with sterile normal saline and dry the canal as before;

(c) pass a fine file (size 20/25) into the canal to the working length and feel for a hard tissue barrier at or around the working length. If a barrier is not present, re-fill the canal with calcium hydroxide as before and arrange to review the patient after a further six months.

If a barrier is present (Fig. 7.6), it is then decided whether the tooth should be permanently root filled at this stage or delayed until another time. A major reason for not placing the definitive root filling is if the tooth is due to be moved orthodontically. Apical resorption of up to 2–3 mm is a fairly common side-effect of orthodontic tooth movement and loss of the hard tissue barrier at this stage will make successful root filling much more difficult and rather defeats the object of the previous conservative management. When the root filling is to be delayed, the canal is re-filled with calcium hydroxide which is replenished every six to eight months until the orthodontic tooth movements have been completed. The definitive root filling may then be carried out—laterally condensed gutta percha and root canal sealer.

Definitive root filling: technique

1. Isolate the tooth.

2. Remove the dressing in the access cavity and the cotton pledget, wash out the calcium hydroxide with sterile normal saline and dry the canal.

3. A master gutta percha cone is placed in the root canal—it is often helpful to place the cone into the canal 'thick end first' (Fig. 7.7)—and measured to ensure that it is going all the way in up to the hard tissue barrier.

4. Withdraw the master cone, fill the canal with root canal sealer, coat the master cone with root canal sealer and gently 'puddle it' up into the canal until it reaches the barrier.

5. Complete the root filling using secondary cones condensed laterally to seal the canal in all its dimensions.

6. Remove excess gutta percha and root canal sealant and seal the access cavity with a non-eugenol-containing cement.
7. Take a post-operative radiograph to confirm the adequacy of the root filling (Fig. 7.8).
8. Monitor the tooth at yearly intervals or such intervals that coincide with the patient's regular dental check-up visits.

Variations of the technique

A number of variations of the technique have been described over the years particularly with regard to the medicament(s) used as the root canal dressing. However, the extensive work of Cvek has shown that calcium hydroxide alone is effective in controlling infection in the root canal and allowing periapical healing with apical barrier formation, and it is this method that we recommend on the basis of present knowledge.

As has already been pointed out, systemic antibiotics may be needed, in conjunction with physical drainage, to help control acute infection. There is evidence, albeit inconclusive, that some patients who have been prescribed systemic antibiotics at the same time as the canal was obturated with calcium hydroxide have had accelerated apical barrier formation. However, more work is needed before the routine prescription of antibiotics can be recommended as an adjunct to the calcium hydroxide treatment.

A fairly recent development in the placement of the definitive root filling in immature teeth is the use of hot gutta percha which can be injected into the root canal using a specially designed 'hot-glue gun' One potential hazard is the damage that can be caused to the cementum if the increase in temperature is too high when the gutta percha is injected into the canal. If the cementum becomes necrotic there is a possibility of either external root resorption or replacement root resorption, both or which are slow and result in an ankylosis or, if there is residual infection in the root canal, inflammatory resorption which can be very rapid.

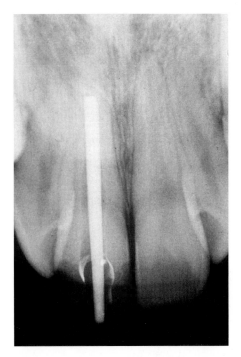

Fig. 7.7 Radiograph of 11 with master gutta percha cone within the root canal, 'thick end first' against the apical barrier.

MODES OF HEALING

Four modes of healing have been described:

1. That shown in Figs 7.8, 7.9, where there is a radiographically identifiable barrier at the apex is found in about 50% of successfully treated teeth.
2. A further variant is when the calcific barrier forms within the canal, coronal to the apex (Figs 7.10, 7.11)—this often results when the calcium hydroxide fails to reach the apex.
3. A third variation is the formation of a barrier which is detectable clinically but is not identifiable radiographically (Figs 7.12, 7.13).
4. The least common is where there has been continued development of the root to give a near normal appearance of the apical aspect of the root (Figs 7.14, 7.15).

THE NATURE OF THE APICAL BARRIER

The presence of an apical barrier impenetrable to a fine endodontic file is the clinical sign that healing has taken place, although the barrier may not always be evident radiographically.

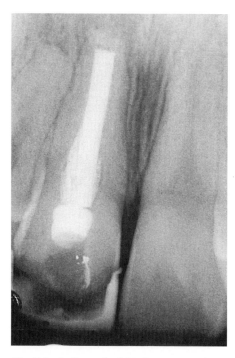

Fig. 7.8 Radiograph of 11 showing completed root filling: laterally condensed multiple gutta percha points and root canal sealer.

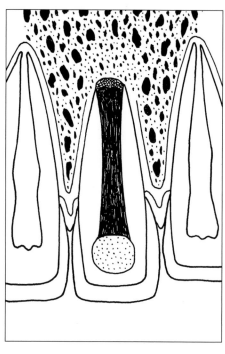

Fig. 7.9 Schematic representation of healing type (1) with the calcific barrier formed at the apex.

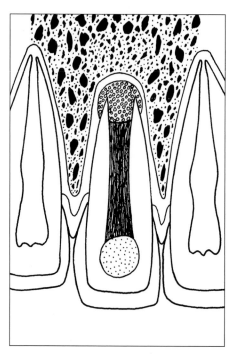

Fig. 7.10 Schematic representation of healing type (2) with the calcific barrier short of the apex within the root canal.

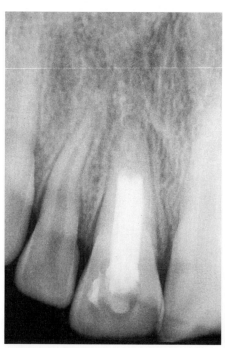

Fig. 7.11 Radiograph of 11 showing healing type (2) with root filling to the barrier within the root canal.

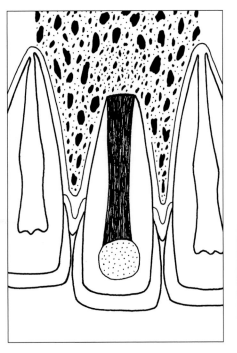

Fig. 7.12 Schematic representation of healing type (3) with the calcific barrier again at the apex but not identifiable radiographically.

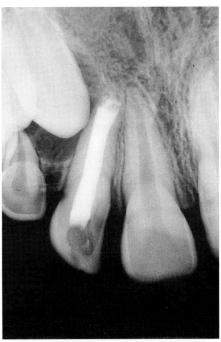

Fig. 7.13 Radiograph of 12 showing healing type (3) with root filling at the apex but no radiographically demonstrable calcific barrier.

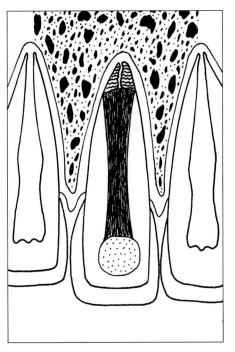

Fig. 7.14 Schematic representation of healing type (4) where there has been continued root formation resulting in an almost normal appearance of the apical aspect of the root.

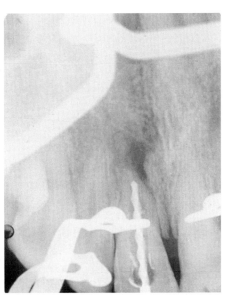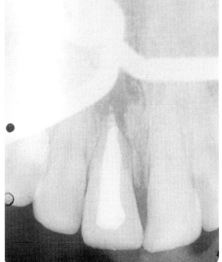

Fig. 7.15 Radiographs of 11 showing healing type (4) where there has been continued root formation at the apex.

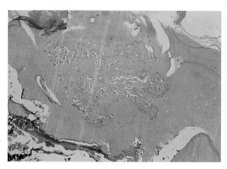

Fig. 7.17 Photomicrograph of the calcific barrier show in Fig. 7.16 at higher magnification. The barrier is formed of cementum and amorphous areas of calcified tissue.

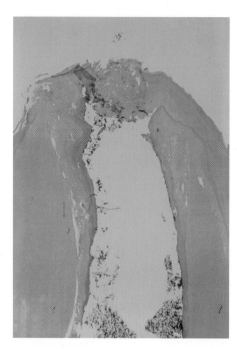

Fig. 7.16 Photomicrograph of a calcific barrier formed at the apex of an upper permanent central incisor which was subsequently lost as the result of further trauma.

The composition of the apical barrier is probably quite variable. As most teeth treated in the prescribed way remain in the patient's mouth for many years they are not often available for histological examination. However, a small number of teeth undergo further trauma which is sufficiently serious for the tooth to be extracted. Examination of specimens obtained in this way (Fig. 7.16) and from primate models show that the apical barrier consists of newly formed cementum and amorphous areas of calcified tissue (Fig. 7.17). The new cementum spans the gap between the walls of the root canal, may grow into the root canal itself appearing to be firmly attached to the dentine, and also appears to be attached to the outer surfaces of the root. Within the hard tissue barrier are areas of connective tissue that are usually non-inflamed. The calcified areas have coarsely granular centres with homogeneous light and dark bands probably associated with calcification of necrotic tissue and have similarities with those seen in the dental pulp following calcium hydroxide pulpotomy. Whatever its true nature, the apical barrier is sufficiently firmly attached to resist the pressures produced during lateral condensation of the root filling.

FACTORS AFFECTING BARRIER FORMATION

Infection within the root canal

Although it has sometimes been suggested that the necrotic pulp tissue in many of these non-vital immature teeth is sterile, careful studies have shown that virtually all are infected with a polymicrobial population of oral commensals. It is possible that these organisms gain access to the root canal from the bloodstream or the gingival crevice either during the period of irreversible pulpitis immediately prior to the pulp becoming necrotic or they infect the pulp after it has become non-vital. Failure to control the infection within the root canal adequately will either increase the time taken for apical healing and barrier formation or actually prevent it.

Root maturity

The rate of barrier formation has been shown to be positively correlated with the state of maturity of the root assessed from the size of the apical foramen, measured radiographically and the age of the patient. The larger the apical foramen or the younger the patient the greater the time taken for apical repair and barrier formation. The difference has been shown to be as much as six months between 8- and 15-year-old children.

Size of the apical radiolucency

Among the changes most commonly associated with necrotic and infected pulp tissue in a root canal is rarefaction of the bone in the vicinity of the apex of the tooth. The endodontic treatment of non-vital immature permanent teeth and the placement of a provisional calcium hydroxide root filling usually results in resolution of these periapical changes associated with infection and the formation of a hard tissue barrier at the apex of the tooth. However, some studies suggest that complete resolution of the apical radiolucency is not required for the apical barrier to form satisfactorily.

COMPLICATIONS

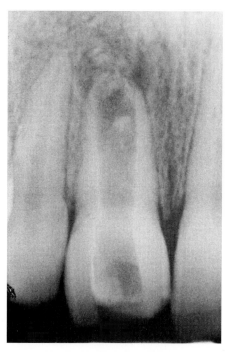

Fig. 7.18 Radiograph of 11 showing incomplete calcific barrier formation.

Escape of calcium hydroxide paste into the periapical tissues

The calcium hydroxide pastes used to obturate the canals of non-vital immature teeth are usually quite soft. The pastes can, therefore, occasionally escape from the confines of the tooth into the periapical tissues during filling of the canal. Although the pH of such pastes is very high they rarely appear to cause any clinical symptoms under such circumstances and are usually readily resorbed from the periapical region.

Incomplete barrier formation

Although clinical assessment of the integrity of the apical barrier is usually carried out with a very fine endodontic file, some barriers may, nevertheless, not be completely solid. Extrusion of root canal sealer into the periapical tissues during root filling is seen from time to time, apparently through very small defects in the apical barrier (Figs 7.18, 7.19). At first sight, the result looks a little untidy but these teeth are found to have as good a prognosis as those with an apparently perfect root filling.

Cystic change

A rare complication in the management of the non-vital immature permanent tooth is the development of a periapical cyst. An apparently routine treatment (Fig. 7.20) had proceeded extremely slowly and the apical radiolucency failed to resolve. Comparison of serial radiographs suggested, in fact, that it had increased in size (Fig. 7.21). Although the barrier had formed it was incomplete and it was anticipated that the sealer would be extruded into the periapical tissues when the tooth was root filled. Arrangements were made, therefore, to carry out an apicectomy and retrograde root filling (Figs 7.22, 7.23).

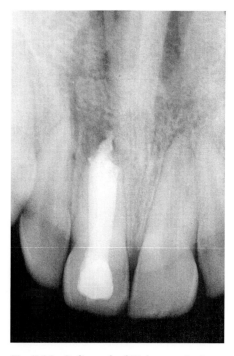

Fig. 7.19 Radiograph of 11 (same patient as in Fig. 7.18) after completion of root filling showing extrusion of small amounts of root canal sealer through defects in the incomplete apical barrier.

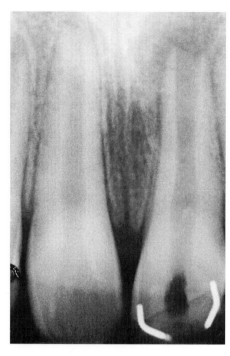

Fig. 7.20 Radiograph of 21 showing persistent periapical infection and bone loss despite calcium hydroxide therapy.

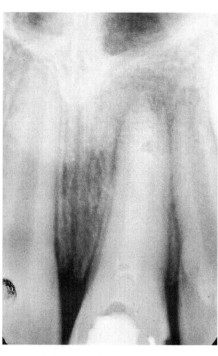

Fig. 7.21 Radiograph of 21 (same patient as Fig. 7.20) showing canal obturated with calcium hydroxide and debatable resolution of apical infection.

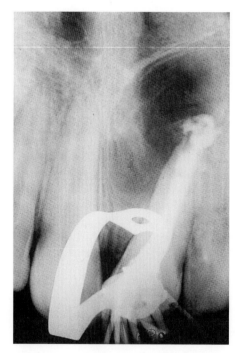

Fig. 7.22 Radiograph of 21 (same patient as Figs 7.20, 7.21) at the time of completion of the permanent root filling.

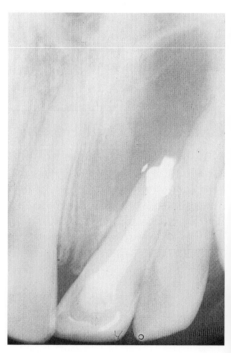

Fig. 7.23 Radiograph of 21 (same patient as in Figs 7.20–7.22) following apical surgery and a retrograde amalgam filling.

FURTHER READING

Cvek, M. (1972). Treatment of non-vital permanent incisors with calcium hydroxide. I. Follow up of periapical repair and apical closure of immature roots. *Odontologisk Revy*, **23**, 27–44.

Frank, A. L. (1966). Therapy for the divergent pulpless tooth by continued apical formation. *Journal of the American Dental Association*, **72**, 87–90.

Gutmann, J. L. and Heaton, J. F. (1981). Management of the open (immature) apex. 2. Non-vital teeth. *International Endodontology Journal*, **14**, 173–7.

Mackie, I. C., Bentley, E. M., and Worthington, H. V., (1988). The closure of open apices in non-vital immature incisor teeth. *British Dental Journal*, **165**, 169–73.

Yates, J. (1988). Barrier formation time in non-vital teeth with open apices. *International Endodontology Journal*, **21**, 313–19.

8   Damage to supporting tissues

8   Damage to supporting tissues

Apart from the periodontal ligament itself the soft tissues frequently involved in oro-dental injury are those of the face, lips, gingivae, alveolar mucosa, frenal attachments, soft palate, and tongue. The most common site for soft tissue injury has been shown to be the lower lip.

Epidemiology

An estimation of the number of soft tissue injuries is extremely difficult. As has been pointed out previously, many oro-dental injuries heal leaving no sign and this is especially true of injuries to the soft tissue in young patients. Rapid healing of minor bruises, abrasions, and cuts, is the norm, so that the great majority of soft tissue injuries are never recorded in epidemiological studies. Also, when there is an associated hard tissue injury, soft tissue injury may go unrecorded or be accorded less attention unless severe. Another factor is that only those injuries considered by the parents to be sufficiently serious to warrant attention result in the child being brought to the dentist or hospital casualty department.

Classification

Injury of the facial and oral soft tissues can be divided into three types: *contusion*, *abrasion*, and *laceration*, with *penetrating wounds* as a separate, fourth, category.

1. Contusion

Damage to the soft tissues results in swelling and bruising (Fig. 8.1) The tissues commonly affected are the attached gingivae and alveolar mucosa labial to the upper central incisors (Fig. 8.2). The bruising and swelling is at a maximum at 48 hours after the accident. The presence of contusion may indicate indirect trauma elsewhere, for example, a bruise on the chin should prompt careful examination of the mandibular condyles.

2. Abrasion

The surface of the affected tissue is lost by being scraped across a rough or uneven surface (e.g. a playground or road) (Fig. 8.3). The surface most commonly affected in this type of injury is that of the face (Fig. 8.4).

3. Laceration

Damage is caused by a solid object cutting through the soft tissues (Fig. 8.5). The cut can be caused by any hard, sharp, object including the patient's own teeth.

Soft tissue injuries frequently present with features of all the above three categories and many lacerations are associated with swelling as the cut is rarely the

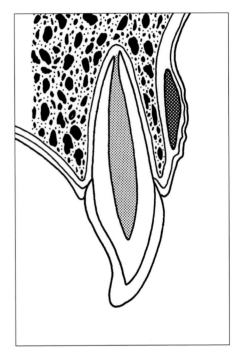

Fig. 8.1   Schematic representation of submucosal bleeding and oedema following injury to the soft tissue overlying the labial surface of the teeth.

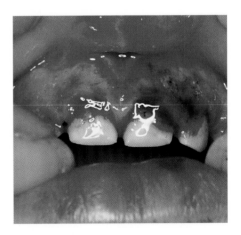

Fig. 8.2   Contusion and abrasion of the soft tissues associated with the labial aspect of the upper deciduous incisors following a fall.

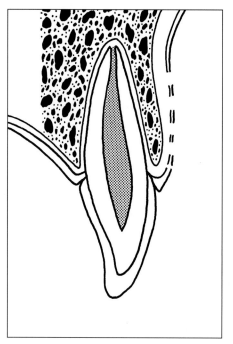

Fig. 8.3 Schematic representation of the effect of abrasion injury on the labial aspect of the soft tissue in the upper incisor region.

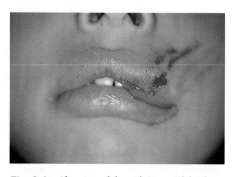

Fig. 8.4 Abrasion of the soft tissue of the face affecting the upper lip and cheek. (There is also a laceration of the upper lip on the same side.

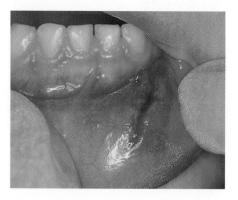

Fig. 8.5 Laceration of the lower lip caused by the patient's teeth when the child ran into another child while playing.

result of a clean 'incision' but a combination of crushing and tearing of the tissue.

4. Penetrating wounds

These are usually produced by a sharp object. This might be the patient's own teeth, a stick or pencil held between the teeth or held by a third party, or a projectile.

Treatment

There seems to be a surprising diversity of views on the management of soft tissue injuries, particularly lacerations and even more particularly, lacerations affecting the tongue. However, there do seem to be some basic principles which should enable decisions to be made that are in the best overall interests of the child or young patient.

The first will be to ensure that there is cessation of bleeding. In fact, by the time most patients attend a dental surgeon, the problem will usually have been resolved by the action of natural haemostatic mechanisms. Dirty wounds of any type should be carefully debrided and washed with a suitable antiseptic solution, and where a gaping wound remains, the edges should be approximated by simple suturing. Where soft tissue has been lost in the accident, referral to a specialist with plastic surgery skills is advisable.

Local considerations

Contusions

These usually only require reassurance and, perhaps, advice on the use of analgesics. For children up to the age of 12 years the analgesic of choice is paracetamol, either sugar-free elixir or tablets. Aspirin should be avoided because of the risk of Reye's syndrome. After the age of 12 years, paracetamol or aspirin may be recommended. Facial bruising may be indicative of secondary trauma elsewhere to the jaws and care should be taken to extend the clinical examination to include all possible sites of secondary trauma.

Abrasions

Abrasions resulting from injury on dirty surfaces should be carefully cleaned with 1% cetrimide or 0.2% chlorhexidene solution to ensure that all grit and other foreign bodies forced into the tissues are washed clear, to minimize the risk of a tattoo. The wounded area may subsequently be very uncomfortable and the temptation to scratch or rub it may be too great for a small child to resist. This discomfort can be alleviated by applying a 1% sodium hydrocortisone ointment three or four times a day for a few days. Large areas of excoriated tissue may require the additional covering of a lint dressing. An alternative to hydrocortisone cream is sterile paraffin wax or petroleum jelly. Analgesics may be also be recommended.

Lacerations

The decision as to whether a laceration should be sutured or not can be difficult. In general, suturing has the advantage that it will reduce the time taken for healing, reduce pain and discomfort during healing, and lead to rapid restoration of soft tissue contour. Against this has to be weighed the additional distress that may be caused by the suturing procedure. If the wound gapes during normal

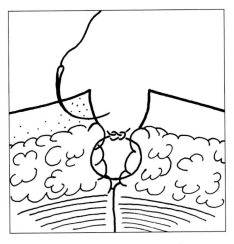

Fig. 8.6 Schematic representation of suturing a deep laceration. A deep suture has already been placed and the superficial tissue is about to be closed.

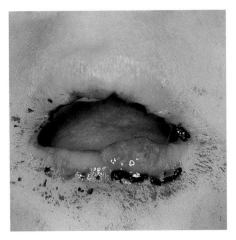

Fig. 8.7 Failure to suture a small laceration of the lower lip has allowed herniation of the underlying soft tissues. There was delayed healing and additional discomfort.

movement or function, suturing is advisable. Very deep lacerations will need closing by placing a deep suture first followed by closure of the more superficial tissues (Fig. 8.6). In the case shown in Fig. 8.7, failure to suture the rather small wound has resulted in the underlying soft tissue herniating through the wound, leading to slower healing and increased discomfort. If the wound stays closed during normal movement and function, and it is felt that suturing would cause undue further distress, the rapid healing usually found, particularly in younger patients, may be relied on to provide a satisfactory outcome.

Penetrating wounds

These may originate from within the oral cavity as, for example, when caused by the patient's own teeth (Fig. 8.5). They may also originate externally, as shown in Fig. 8.8. The child fell over and the stick he was holding between his teeth was forced back into his mouth puncturing the soft palate. The wound was sutured with resorbable suture material (4/0 softgut) under general anaesthesia. As a precaution, the child was kept in hospital overnight because of the possible risk of airway obstruction caused by further, post-operative swelling of the damaged soft tissues. A foreign body may also enter the lip from the external surface. The wound in the lip in Fig. 8.9 was thought to have been caused by a ricochet from an air-gun, which was confirmed on the lateral radiograph (Fig. 8.10). To reduce the risk of serious damage to the labial artery an incision was made along the line of the lip, and *not* transversely, the air-gun pellet was then removed (Fig. 8.11). The superficial and surgical access was closed with 4/0 black silk and the wound healed uneventfully.

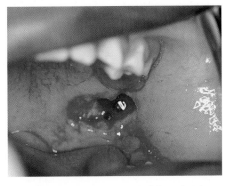

Fig. 8.8 Penetrating wound of the soft palate, caused by the child falling on to a stick held between his teeth.

Laceration of the tongue

From time to time the tongue is bitten during a fall, especially in small children. Tongue lacerations are technically difficult to suture adequately and the sutures are frequently lost within a day or so of placement. As many injuries of this type are to small children, the suturing may often only be achieved under general anaesthesia or sometimes local analgesia with inhalation sedation as an adjunct. Many tongue lacerations heal with remarkable rapidity without treatment. Some, however, heal more slowly, usually when the wound gapes widely, the healing then being by secondary rather than primary intention and residual scarring may result. These factors lead a number of clinicians to doubt the necessity for

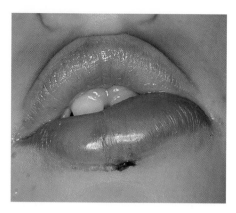

Fig. 8.9 Penetrating wound of the lip from the external surface caused by the ricochet of an air-gun pellet.

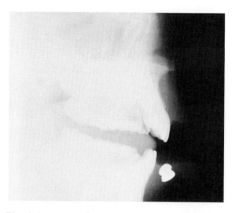

Fig. 8.10 Lateral radiograph of the patient in Fig. 8.9 showing the foreign body in the lower lip.

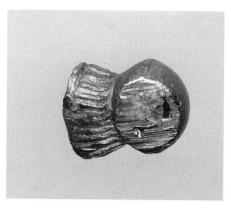

Fig. 8.11 Air-gun pellet removed from the lower lip of the patient in Figs 8.9, 8.10.

suturing tongue lacerations. The authors feel that as lacerations in general heal more quickly when sutured, tongue lacerations should be similarly treated but only if the sutures are able to be placed properly with the expectation that they will be retained long enough for healing by primary intention—probably 3 to 5 days.

Most patients with contusions, abrasions, and simple lacerations may be cared for by their general dental practitioner but any patient with a wound requiring more extensive care should be referred to a specialist with plastic surgery skills.

BONY TISSUES

Injury to the teeth and/or soft tissues usually also results in damage to the associated bone. This is frequently not serious and requires no special treatment. The minimum injury is probably some bruising and comminution of the internal surface of the alveolus of an affected tooth. At the other extreme, are fractures which can involve the bones of the facial skeleton, including the body of the mandible, the condylar neck, zygomatic process, and maxilla. The management of fractures of the facial skeleton are outside the scope of this book. However, it is important that the general dental practitioner is familiar with the principles of the diagnosis and first aid care for patients with such injury. For example, a patient who attends, following injury, with a mildly bruised chin, but also complains of pain in the pre-auricular area on one side may have damaged the condyle on the other side. Clinical examination will reveal that the patient deviates noticeably to one side on opening. This is typical of a fracture of the neck of the condyle on the side to which the patient deviates. Conservative management is usually adopted in such cases:

(a) reassurance;

(b) encouragement of normal jaw movement;

(c) a soft diet;

(d) analgesics.

Interference with the growth centre of the mandibular condyle is, fortunately, an extremely rare complication in such cases. The condylar head, neck, and associated glenoid fossa undergo varying degrees of remodelling and long-term functional disturbance of the temporo-mandibular joint is also extremely unusual.

Epidemiology

As with soft tissue injuries, the true prevalence of bone fractures is difficult to estimate. Many of the minor injuries go unrecorded—for example, the minor fractures of the alveolar process associated with luxation injuries are usually of little consequence and heal rapidly. Nevertheless, it has been shown that fractures of the jaw in children constitute approximately 10% of all fractures involving the facial skeleton. The most common site for bony fractures is the condylar neck followed by the body of the mandible (Table 8.1). The majority of these are the result of incidents involving considerable force (e.g. road traffic accidents and falls from a height).

FURTHER READING

Andreasen, J. O. and Andreasen, F. M. (1994). *Textbook and color atlas of traumatic injuries to the teeth*, (3rd edn), pp. 495–516. Munksgaard, Copenhagen.

Keniry, A. J. (1971). A survey of jaw fractures in children. *British Journal of Oral Surgery*, **8**, 231–6.

Sahm, G. and Witt, E. (1989) Long-term results after childhood condylar fractures. A computer-tomographic study. *European Journal of Orthodontics*, **11**, 154–60.

Table 8.1 Jaw fractures in children

Type	n	%
Symphysis	5	6.2
Body of mandible	30	37.1
Ramus (including coronoid and angle)	4	4.9
Unilateral subcondylar	17	21.0
Bilateral subcondylar	12	14.8
Alveolar fractures (including premaxilla)	12	14.8
Zygomatic arch	1	1.2
Total	81	100

Note: the bilateral subcondylar figure of 12 represents 24 fractures in 12 patients.
After Keniry (1971).

Index